Your Roadmap to Successful Asthma Treatment

Your Roadmap to Successful Asthma Treatment

Joi S. Lucas, MD

YOUR ROADMAP TO SUCCESSFUL ASTHMA TREATMENT
Copyright © 2021 Joi S. Lucas
All rights reserved.

Published by Publish Your Gift®
An imprint of Purposely Created Publishing Group, LLC

Printed in the United States of America

ISBN: 978-1-64484-371-0 (print)
ISBN: 978-1-64484-372-7 (ebook)

Special discounts are available on bulk quantity purchases by book clubs, associations and special interest groups. For details email: sales@publishyourgift.com or call (888) 949-6228. For information log on to www.PublishYourGift.com

Table of Contents

Acknowledgments

To my coach and mentor, Dr. Draion Burch,
thank you for your encouragement and wisdom.

Thank you to my mother and Shero,
Dr. Sheryl Guthrie Lucas Giles,
for blazing the trail while inspiring me to dream big,
achieve, and keep my eyes on the prize.

To my father, Theodore Lucas,
thank you for making me strong and a little stubborn.

Mike and Maurice, the best brothers ever,
thanks for all of the adventures.

To Careina, Bettina, and Andrea,
Thanks for your lifelong friendship and excellent advice.

For my husband, Frank A. Jones,
a tremendous thank you for your
unconditional love and support.

Introduction
So Your Child Has Asthma?

When your child is diagnosed with asthma, the basics of breathing are challenged. You question how did this happen, and what can I do to make this better? Is all of this medicine really necessary? Whether you are a parent, grandparent, teacher, or caregiver, you may feel overwhelmed and uncertain about the diagnosis and treatment options offered. As a lung specialist for children or pediatric pulmonologist, I have cared for thousands of kids with asthma, and my goal is to improve their quality of life. As a lifelong asthmatic, I understand how asthma can deprive you of precious time and the simple joys of health some take for granted. To effectively treat childhood asthma, taking prescribed medicines is simply not enough. You need a clear, organized, and decisive roadmap specific to your child's needs. As a parent, your power is knowing your child better than anyone, and your mission is getting the right help for your child. As a grandparent, teacher, or caregiver, you must be well-informed. The missing link to controlling asthma is understanding the disease. This book gives you straightforward information and the strategies needed to attain your goal and to successfully treat your child's asthma with the right medications. It is organized by commonly asked questions about asthma. You do not have to read the chapters in order; feel free to skip to the burning question you want answered first for your child. I have included medical terms with a definition, so you are not confused by "doctor talk" when you have your doctor's appointment. There are expert tips throughout the book, giving you helpful hints that are important to learn if you are short on time and cannot read the entire chapter. All parents, kids, and people who have asthma can benefit from reading this book. However, I have a special interest in helping parents and caregivers of children with recently diagnosed asthma, uncontrolled symptoms, or those looking for an off ramp from use of long-term medications. I understand the daily struggle of dealing with asthma and endeavor to prescribe (and take) the least medications possible with the best results.

The information provided is meant to complement the assessment and instructions provided by your doctor and is not in any way an independent method to diagnose or treat asthma. Your doctor is your trusted partner in caring for *your* child with asthma. However, in any great partnership, you must bring something valuable to the table. Reading this book enables you to be an optimal partner with your doctor, both by broadening your understanding of asthma and revealing your doctor's process for treating your child. COVID-19 and the global pandemic have upended our daily lives. Now is the time for you to proactively navigate your child's asthma diagnosis and treatment in a post-pandemic world.

How Do the Lungs Work?

The lungs are the primary place where asthma happens. They are a pair of spongy, air-filled sacs (or organs) in the chest, along with the heart, great blood vessels, and other structures. The main job of the lungs is to deliver oxygen from the air we breathe to the bloodstream.

When you inhale air, it first enters the nose. Breathing through your nose instead of your mouth naturally protects you from viruses and bacteria. The nose is the gateway to the respiratory tract and specifically designed to defend the airway. Air breathed through the nose is warmed, moistened, and filtered to prevent pathogens such as viruses, fungi, bacteria, and pollutants from entering the upper respiratory tract. The nasal lining produces mucus trapping particles and immune cells deployed to actively fight infection. Air then passes through the nasal canals into the throat and past the larynx (voice box) which houses the vocal cords. When air passes over the vocal cords, they vibrate, producing sounds and allowing speech. Air then flows to the trachea or windpipe. The trachea is located in front of the esophagus, the major tube leading to the stomach.

The lungs are shaped like an inverted tree with the trachea dividing into left and right bronchi. In fact, we call the airway branches the bronchial tree. One branch is a bronchus, and the plural are bronchi. There are sections in the lungs called lobes. In each of the lobes, the bronchi divide

3

several times until reaching the bronchioles or small airways. Bronchi and bronchioles have an airway lining and a muscle wrapping around the outside of the tube. The bronchioles end in alveoli, tiny air sacs, where vital oxygen is delivered to the bloodstream in exchange for carbon dioxide, the waste gas exhaled out of the body. When oxygen moves from the alveoli into the bloodstream, it leaves the lungs and is carried by the blood vessels to the heart. The heart is the body's engine which pumps blood and oxygen to the rest of the organs. You might think of oxygen as fuel for the body, just as gasoline is fuel for a car.

Grasping the basic mechanics of breathing allows you to determine if your child is breathing well or having difficulty. Knowing this moves you further toward your goal of controlling your child's asthma. The diaphragm is the major muscle of respiration and is located mid-chest, below the lungs. When you inhale, it moves lower in the chest and outward, allowing the lungs to expand and draw in air. Between the ribs are the intercostal muscles that when contracted pull the ribs upwards and outward, increasing the size of the chest cavity. The chest wall and the lungs are elastic. Exhalation or breathing out is passive, and airflow out of the lungs happens when the lungs and chest wall recoil.

When infants and children have difficulty breathing, they retract or use additional muscles to open the airway. Doctors call this breathing "respiratory distress." Retractions of the lungs appear as abdominal breathing, pulling in of the chest underneath the rib cage, pulling of intercostal muscles, and a depression at the base of the neck. Tachypnea or fast respiratory rate is a sensitive sign of respiratory distress in infants and young children. Nasal flaring or expanding of the nostrils is also a sign that your child is having difficulty breathing. Normal breathing or respiratory rates vary with the age of the child. Make sure you check with your doctor to know what a normal respiratory rate or amount of breaths per minute is for their age.

Expert Tip

Observing what your child's chest looks like while breathing normally is critical to knowing if he or she is breathing abnormally when sick.

What Is Asthma?

Asthma is a lung condition causing recurring symptoms of shortness of breath, chest tightness, cough, and wheezing or whistling of the airway. In the United States (US), asthma is the leading chronic or long-lasting, childhood illness with over ten million children and teenagers diagnosed. When you have asthma, swelling in the airway lining of the bronchi and bronchioles produces thick mucus plugging up the airways. Bronchoconstriction or tightening of the airway muscle decreases airflow. Children with asthma may have symptoms such as breathlessness, difficulty exercising, chest pain, fatigue, pallor, blue lips and face, sighing, or an inability to speak in full sentences. Asthmatics can have a productive (wet) or dry cough. Some children with asthma may be asymptomatic or have no symptoms for long periods of time. Sudden onset of symptoms is called an asthma attack. If asthma goes untreated, a structural change may develop with thickening or remodeling of the airways. Treating asthma prevents loss of lung function and reduced lung growth.

Triggers are environmental exposures causing asthma symptoms and can be different for every child. Common triggers for asthma symptoms are strong odors (i.e., bleach or cleaning supplies), tobacco smoke, allergy to dust mite (microscopic insect like pests feeding off of skin cells), pollen, animals (cat, dog), cockroaches, mold, temperature change, heat, humidity, exercise, emotion, pollution, and viral illness. Avoiding known triggers for asthma is important to maintaining control of your child's asthma. An asthma attack or exacerbation occurs when asthmatics are exposed to a trigger and respiratory symptoms suddenly worsen due to closure of the airways. Respiratory distress during an asthma attack is life-threatening, and children can die from severe asthma symptoms. Asthma is the leading cause of emergency department visits and hospitalizations for US children. Early recognition of asthma symptoms helps prevent asthma attacks and complications.

The exact mechanism for development of asthma is unknown. It is thought to involve the interaction between genetics (heredity) and environmental exposures occurring during critical stages of immune system development. There have been many studies associating asthma with certain characteristics you should know. Children with asthma are more likely to have one of the following:

- elevated body mass index (BMI) or be overweight,
- low birth weight,
- formula fed,
- male gender,
- family history of asthma,
- live with a smoker,
- family income below the poverty line,
- attend day care,
- African American or Puerto Rican descent.

Other major risk factors for asthma include sensitization (allergic or immune reaction) to house dust mite, alternaria (mold), and viral respiratory infections (respiratory syncytial virus (RSV) and rhinovirus).

There are two major inflammatory pathways suspected to produce asthma. The first pathway causes activation of allergy cells such as eosinophils, mast cells, and basophils which increase levels of immunoglobulin E (IgE), an antibody or part of the immune system generating allergic response. IgE stimulates allergic asthma by causing mucus hyperproduction, airway obstruction, airway muscle hypertrophy (enlargement) in the bronchi/bronchioles, airway hyperreactivity (triggered airway closure), and structural remodeling. In this type of allergic asthma, there is also elevated nitric oxide, a gas given off by a swollen airway lining with lots of eosinophils. This first asthma pathway produces a type of asthma called type 2 (T2) high asthma. The second major asthma pathway is called T2 low asthma and is driven by neutrophils, an immune cell fighting infection. In T2 low asthma, there are normal levels of eosinophils in blood and airway mucus. Most asthma medications currently available are directed toward T2 high asthma or more allergic asthma.

One theory of how asthma originates is called the "hygiene hypothesis" and proposes that our modern environment is very clean, too clean. Reduced exposure to germs and the outdoors prevents the immune system from learning to recognize true invaders such as viruses and bacteria from harmless exposures. This creates a supercharged immune system that sensitizes children to allergens. This model is supported by findings that for instance, living on a farm is associated with a 23 percent reduced chance of asthma. However, to date, the science behind this is not definitively proven or universally accepted. I moved to Des Moines, Iowa, for three years and unfortunately, this did not resolve my asthma symptoms.

Asthma is likely inherited through a complex process comprising multiple genes. This makes it hard to predict who will have asthma. However, if a parent has asthma, their child is almost twice as likely to have asthma as someone with no family history. If parents and grandparents have asthma, a child may be four times more likely to have asthma. Before puberty, boys are more prone to asthma compared to girls and twice as likely as girls to be hospitalized for an asthma exacerbation. Young boys have a smaller airway diameter relative to lung volume when compared to girls, increasing the risk for asthma morbidity. After puberty, asthma is more common in girls. During adolescence, there is a decline in the severity of asthma illness in males compared to females.

There is no cure for asthma, but there are excellent treatments that work for most patients. Regular follow-ups with your doctor are important for keeping your child with asthma healthy. Keep reading, and I'll explain more to get you ready for your doctor's visit.

Does My Child Have Asthma?

There are clear guidelines for asthma diagnosis that were developed over twenty years ago and recommendations for treatment updated in 2020. However, arriving at a definitive diagnosis of asthma can still be difficult. Many parents do not recognize their child's symptoms as an indication they have asthma.

A diagnosis of asthma is made by evaluating patterns of respiratory symptoms over time that limit breathing and for children over five years of age, the completion of a breathing test is required. These questions will help you determine if your child has asthma:

- Does your child cough or wheeze apart from colds?
- How often is coughing present? Once per day, multiple times per day, one to two times per week?
- Does the cough produce mucus or sputum?
- Is there coughing or wheezing overnight?
- Do the symptoms vary in intensity?
- Has your child been to the doctor or emergency department for their breathing?
- Has your child missed school because of his or her symptoms?
- Does your child need albuterol for difficulty breathing?

- Does asthma run in your family?
- Does your child have allergies or eczema?
- Has your child been hospitalized for difficulty breathing?
- Has your child ever needed oral steroids?

The rule of twos is what doctors use to assess if your child's respiratory symptoms make a diagnosis of asthma likely. If your child coughs, wheezes, or has difficulty breathing greater than two times per week, awakens overnight with respiratory symptoms more than two times per month, or needs albuterol more than two times per week apart from activity, they may have asthma.

Asthma is classified as intermittent, mild, moderate, or severe based upon the frequency of symptoms. In young children, a diagnosis of asthma is often made after a trial of asthma medications shows improvement of respiratory symptoms while on medications and worsening once medications are stopped.

Expert Tip

Your job as a parent is not to make a diagnosis of asthma but to recognize when your child is having difficulty breathing. Your doctor will provide guidance on your child's asthma classification.

Intermittent Asthma

Kids with intermittent asthma have symptoms no more than two days per week. Asthma causes no interference with normal activity, and they have normal lung function. Children five and older have nighttime awakenings for asthma symptoms less than two times per month. They need a rescue medicine such as albuterol less than two days per week, excluding use for exercise. They have asthma exacerbations requiring oral steroids no more than one time per year.

Mild Persistent Asthma

These children have symptoms more than two days per week but not daily. Children five and older have nighttime awakenings for asthma three to four times per month; those under five years have nighttime awakenings one to two times per month. They have minor limitation of breathing with activity. Lung function is normal. They need a rescue medication such as albuterol more than two days per week but not daily. For children over five years, oral steroids are needed for asthma exacerbations two or more times per year. Children under five years old have four or more episodes of wheezing lasting more than one day or during the past six months have two or more asthma exacerbations, in addition to risk factors for persistent asthma.

Moderate Persistent Asthma

Children have daily asthma symptoms. Kids five years and older have nighttime awakenings for asthma greater than one night per week but not nightly. Children under five years of age have nighttime awakenings three to four times per month. They have some limitation of breathing with activity. They need a rescue medication such as albuterol daily. Lung function is reduced. Oral steroids are needed for asthma exacerbations two or more times per year.

Severe Persistent Asthma

Children have asthma symptoms throughout the day. Children five years and older have nighttime awakenings for asthma seven times per week, and children under five years of age experience awakenings more than once a week. A rescue medication such as albuterol is needed several times per day. They have extremely limited ability to exercise. Lung function is significantly reduced. Oral steroids are needed for asthma exacerbations two or more times per year. Severe asthmatics represent 5 percent of all childhood asthma cases.

As you can see, making a diagnosis of asthma is no easy task. Many children have symptom severity between two classifications or only have symptoms seasonally. They may be fine during the summer but have severe, persistent asthma symptoms in the fall and winter. Don't worry; your job as a parent is not to make the diagnosis. Providing an excellent history of how and when symptoms happen gives your doctor the information needed to make an accurate diagnosis.

What Tests Can Be Done to Diagnose Asthma?

It is important to confirm a diagnosis of asthma so unnecessary treatment is avoided. Asthma symptoms may come and go, and oftentimes, a symptom like wheezing is not present when you visit the doctor. However, the underlying causes of asthma including airway inflammation and airway narrowing persist, even when no obvious respiratory symptoms are noticed.

For children over five years of age, a breathing test called spirometry may be used to determine if airflow from the lungs is limited by obstruction, and you have asthma. During spirometry testing, your child will be encouraged to blow air out from their lungs into a device measuring how quickly they can empty air from their lungs. An important part of this test is called forced expiratory volume in the first second (FEV1). FEV1 measures how fast your child's lungs can empty air over one second. Healthy lungs can empty 80 percent or more in one second. (The test is based on a scale of 100 percent.) FEV1 has normal ranges that vary based upon age, height, gender, and race. Your child's FEV1 results will be compared to normal results of other kids matching them. If a child's FEV1 is lower than expected, this increases the risk their airway is blocked or obstructed by mucus or inflammation. If lung function improves by 12 percent after taking albuterol, the rescue medication, a diagnosis of asthma can be made. It is important that before the test you do not consume caffeine, which improves lung function for one to two hours, or take medications such as albuterol that will alter test results. More detailed lung function testing can be completed for the diagnosis of exercise induced asthma.

A bronchoprovocation test is a type of lung function test used to diagnose asthma. It works by challenging or irritating the airway with various substances such as histamine (a particle in the body causing allergic response), cold air, exercise, or methacholine, an inhaled drug causing mild airway narrowing. If lung function decreases after exposure to these challenges, a diagnosis of asthma is possible.

A peak expiratory flow (PEF) meter is a handheld device measuring the air pushed out by the lungs. It is dependent on respiratory effort and less reliable than spirometry for diagnosis of asthma. However, it can be used to monitor asthma symptoms. Excessive variability of twice daily PEF over two weeks can be used to show airflow limitations. Keep in mind you should use the same PEF meter. Readings from different PEF devices can vary as much as 20 percent.

Immunoglobulin E (IgE) responds to environmental triggers and plays a major role in allergic response. Asthmatics often have an elevated IgE level. Blood testing for IgE is helpful in the diagnosis of allergic asthma.

Eosinophils are specialized cells of the immune system associated with allergic disorders. A blood eosinophil count greater than 4 percent is suggestive of asthma. Eosinophil levels are included in a complete blood count (CBC) with an extended white blood cell (immune cell) profile, or differential.

Allergy testing identifies environmental and food triggers to avoid and is important in assisting with preventing allergic asthma symptoms. Positive allergy testing alone does not confirm a diagnosis of asthma. Allergy testing may be completed by blood or skin prick.

There are several questionnaires developed to assess asthma symptoms. The Asthma Control Test (ACT) is a popular one that may be administered quickly and has a score indicating risk of uncontrolled asthma.

Fractional concentration of exhaled nitric oxide (FeNO) is a breathing test measuring the amount of nitric oxide present in exhaled air. FeNO is elevated in asthmatics with allergic inflammation. However, it does not reveal asthma in people with non-allergic asthma. FeNO is a helpful tool, assisting in making the diagnosis of asthma.

Chest radiograph (chest x-ray) allows the anatomy (structure) of the lung to be evaluated. It is helpful to also rule out other possible causes of respiratory symptoms such as infection or abnormality causing airway compression.

Flexible bronchoscopy uses a scope (camera entering the airway) to directly visualize the airway and assists with diagnosis of severe asthma. This procedure completed in the operating room (OR) under anesthesia includes a bronchoalveolar lavage (lung washing) to evaluate airway fluid for infection and allergic sensitization.

Will My Child Grow Out of Asthma?

One of the most common questions asked by parents and caregivers is when will a child outgrow asthma. Many adults recall that they had asthma as a child but "outgrew" it. The truth is, whether your asthma symptoms go away or not is based upon a complex interaction of factors that are not fully understood. Some research studies suggest kids who are allergic and have more severe asthma when they are younger tend to have asthma persisting into adulthood. In fact, about one-third of children with asthma will continue to have symptoms when they get older. However, if you have asthma, the symptoms can come back at any point under the right circumstances. For most children, only time will tell if they will be in the group who has lessened symptoms as they get older.

A diagnosis of asthma can be confusing because symptoms are not present all the time, and seasonal variation in severity may happen. Unfortunately, even when asthma symptoms are not noticeable for a while, it does not mean your child has outgrown asthma. Lung function testing (spirometry) for kids five and older is an objective measure of asthma. This test compares how well an asthmatic child's lungs empty air to the expected norms of children without asthma. If your child's lung function is decreased, chances are they have not outgrown asthma. The most important thing to keep in mind is the here and now. If asthma symptoms are present, you should treat them. Children who have poorly controlled or untreated asthma are at risk for reduced lung growth and permanently decreased lung function. If lung function remains normal and no asthma symptoms have been present for several years, then there is a chance your child will be in the group of kids who escape asthma as an adult.

Did My Pregnancy Cause Childhood Asthma?

Genetics are not the only predictor of asthma in children. Lifestyle and health during pregnancy can determine if your child is at higher risk for asthma. Breastfeeding is protective, meaning there is a decreased risk of having asthma if an infant is breastfed during the first three months of life.

Maternal diet matters. Studies have shown that high maternal vitamin D or vitamin E during pregnancy is associated with reduced chance of wheezing in early childhood. Some research reveals increased intake of fruits can significantly reduce the odds of asthma; a Mediterranean diet (rich in fiber, lower in saturated fats, and high in olive or fish oil) also decreased the risk of asthma. There are no reported benefits for mothers who took supplements prenatally like copper, calcium, magnesium, manganese, or selenium. Probiotics during pregnancy are not significantly associated with improvement in asthma risk. Of course, you should take your prenatal vitamin and any other medications recommended by your doctor if you are pregnant.

There is a strong association between maternal obesity and childhood asthma. If a mother is overweight during pregnancy or has elevated body mass index (BMI), there is over 1.2 times increased chance of her child having asthma. In addition, the more overweight a mom is, the stronger the risk for asthma is in her baby. If you are pregnant, make sure you speak with your physician about what a healthy diet and weight are for you.

Use of antibiotics during pregnancy is associated with an increased odds of childhood wheezing or asthma. Specifically, antibiotic use in the third trimester has a stronger association with wheezing or asthma than antibiotic use in the first or second trimester of pregnancy. Acetaminophen use in pregnancy is also associated with a higher risk of childhood asthma.

Prenatal maternal smoking significantly increases the risk of asthma in all age groups but is higher in children under five years of age. Paternal smoking prenatally is also associated with increased risk of asthma.

Cesarean section is associated with increased risk of childhood asthma, and pre-term labor is linked with almost one and a half times increased risk of asthma or wheezing. Specifically, children less than thirty-two weeks gestation and with low birth weight (<2,500g) have a higher risk of asthma. However, children with high birth weight are also at increased risk of developing asthma. Jaundice and the need for phototherapy (lights for high bilirubin) after birth increases the risk of asthma. Maternal stress is also linked to the development of childhood wheezing.

The vast number of risk factors that can increase the chance of childhood asthma illustrate the complexities of the disease process. Some of these risk factors may be out of your control. However, breastfeeding, a healthy diet, controlling weight, quitting smoking, decreasing stress, and not opting for a scheduled cesarean section are all ways to reduce the risk for asthma that you can control.

What Are Some Asthma Myths and Facts?

As an asthmatic myself, I have heard many myths about asthma treatments that are more fiction than fact. Dispelling myths about asthma allows kids and parents to focus on effective ways to manage symptoms and have a great quality of life. Keep reading to see if you have heard any of these common asthma myths.

Myth 1 – Kids with asthma cannot exercise or participate in physical education.

This is not true. Kids with asthma can and should exercise. Regular exercise can help prevent obesity, improve endurance, and increase lung capacity. When asthma symptoms are controlled, kids with asthma can exercise safely. Some kids need to take a bronchodilator or rescue medication like albuterol before activity. If your child wheezes or is extremely tired during exercise, talk to your doctor about the best medications to resolve those symptoms.

Myth 2 – There is a cure for asthma.

Unfortunately, this is not true. There is no cure for asthma; however, there are great medications that can improve symptoms.

Myth 3 – Inhaled steroids are the same as body builder steroids.

No, this is not true. Inhaled or oral corticosteroids used to treat asthma are a different class of medication than anabolic steroids, the type of medications used illegally by athletes to build muscle. Asthma medications will not cause your child to have rippling muscles.

Myth 4 – Kids cannot die from asthma.

Sadly, this is not true. Kids can die from asthma, and adults can too. Boys are more likely to die from asthma than girls. Women are more likely to die of asthma than men. African Americans are three times more likely to die from asthma than people of other races or ethnicities, with African American women having the highest death rates. Most asthma deaths are preventable with the use of medications and the care of a doctor.

Myth 5 – Asthma is in your mind or imagined.

Asthma is real and not imaginary. It is not caused by laziness or lack of effort. Asthma is a condition that cannot be controlled with the mind. Medication is needed to stop the underlying changes in the body that produce asthma symptoms.

Myth 6 – Asthma medications are habit-forming.

Asthma medications are not habit-forming or addictive like opioids or other classes of potentially addictive medications. If your child stops using daily asthma medications, the medication will stop working, and the underlying causes of asthma will return. Make sure you discuss with your doctor when it is safe to stop asthma medications.

Myth 7 – Chihuahuas can cure asthma.

There is a legend that Chihuahuas will take on a child's asthma and cure them of asthma. This is not true. I fully support Chihuahuas as a loving pet. However, they cannot cure asthma in children.

Are Allergies, Eczema, and Asthma Connected?

Atopy is the genetic tendency to develop allergic diseases like asthma, allergic rhinitis (runny nose with sneezing), and eczema, a condition causing red and itchy skin. The allergic triad of asthma, allergies, and eczema is common. Almost 90 percent of asthmatic children show allergic sensitization. Having eczema matters when it comes to a diagnosis of asthma in children. Nearly 13 percent of US children have eczema, and 30 percent of children with eczema develop asthma. Most children with eczema are diagnosed before five years of age. Asthma can be described as eczema of the airway and eczema as asthma of the skin. If your child has eczema, you should be vigilant and aware of respiratory symptoms that may be asthma. In some children, worsened eczema symptoms may precede an asthma exacerbation. The "allergic march" describes a pattern of developing eczema and food allergy early in childhood, turning into asthma and rhinitis or swollen runny nose in later childhood.

Allergy testing either through a skin prick or blood testing is important to understand allergen triggers for asthma. Measuring the blood level of immunoglobulin E (IgE), a part of the immune system associated with allergic response, helps determine the likelihood of atopy in a child. Controlling an allergy symptom like post-nasal drip from allergic rhinitis is important for resolving asthma symptoms. Allergic rhinitis is treated with a nasal corticosteroid spray like fluticasone propionate (Flonase®) or mometasone furoate (Nasonex®) and an antihistamine like cetirizine or loratadine. Allergy sensitization increases the risk for asthma, eczema, and allergies that persist into adulthood.

Food allergy should be ruled out as a possible cause of symptoms. If your child experiences hives, a red itchy skin rash, swelling of the lips/tongue, vomiting, or wheezing after eating certain foods, they could have food allergy. For children with food allergy or moderate to severe environmental allergies, a consultation with an allergist is helpful in determining what to avoid and if your child is eligible for immunotherapy (allergy shots) or other medications. However, if food allergy causes severe cough or wheezing, call 911 immediately and give epinephrine, a life-saving treatment for severe allergic reaction called anaphylaxis.

How Do I Avoid Asthma Triggers?

Avoidance of known asthma triggers is critical to preventing exacerbation of asthma symptoms. By avoiding asthma triggers, you can also lessen the need for medications. For some children, the exact cause of asthma symptoms is a mystery. Common triggers for asthma symptoms include temperature changes, heat, humidity, cold air, exercise, emotions, viral illness, strong odors (i.e., bleach or cleaning supplies), tobacco smoke, allergy to dust mites, pollens, animal dander (skin), cockroaches, and molds. If your child is allergic to pets like cats and dogs, animals should not be allowed in the bedroom, and children should not sleep with the pet. A vacuum with a high-efficiency particulate air (HEPA) filter is recommended for carpet. In some instances, the pet may need to be removed from the home.

Expert Tip

Before you remove a pet from the home because they are suspected to cause asthma and allergy symptoms, make sure you have your child tested for allergies.

In children with dust mite allergy, washing bedding and stuffed animals in hot water weekly, vacuuming carpet frequently, in addition to using special mite-proof mattress and pillow covers is recommended. Stuffed animals should not be kept on the bed because they can collect dust. Keeping the humidity in your home low will also help control dust mites. If you live in a home or apartment with water damage, mold could be a trigger for asthma symptoms. Remediating or fixing mold growth is important. Changing air conditioner filters at least once per month is recommended to prevent aeroallergens (allergens in the air). Air purifiers may be helpful in homes with indoor smoke exposure or significant pet dander (skin flakes). Controlling pests like roaches and mice will reduce the risk of this causing asthma symptoms. If your child has tree, weed, or grass allergies, make sure you limit outdoor activity during the season when pollen from the offending plant is present.

Smoking or vaping outside of the home and car is critical and quitting smoking/vaping is the best option for caregivers of children with asthma. Most of the patients I see in my office for asthma have a smoker in the family. Second-hand smoke exposure is a strong trigger for asthma symptoms. Caregivers who are smokers or who vape should wear a smoking jacket and hat to cover their hair. After smoking, they should change their shirt and wash their face and hands. Teens with asthma cannot smoke or vape.

What Is Exercise Induced Asthma?

Exercise is one of the most common triggers for asthma symptoms in children. Exercise induced bronchoconstriction (EIB) is narrowing of the airway that occurs with exercise. Children typically experience chest tightness, shortness of breath, cough, wheezing, or difficulty breathing specifically with exercise. The exact cause of EIB is unknown but is suspected to occur when cells causing inflammation are released in the airway. In addition, large volumes of cold, dry air inhaled into the airway causes rapid loss of the heat and water from the airway lining, leading to bronchoconstriction or airway narrowing. If a clear diagnosis of EIB is in doubt, an exercise challenge test may confirm a decrease in lung function, forced expiratory volume in the first second (FEV1) after exercise. Children run on a treadmill or ride a bike while breathing dry air, and serial lung function testing is completed. If there is a fall in lung function (FEV1) by a certain percentage from normal, the test shows exercise induced asthma. Alternatives to exercise testing have been developed for diagnosis of EIB in children using other methods such as mannitol (dry powder), dry air, or concentrated salt water (hypertonic saline). An exercise test or indirect challenge test for most kids is not needed. Children and their parents simply report shortness of breath or wheezing specifically with activity that is alleviated by rest or use of an albuterol inhaler.

> ### *Expert Tip*
>
> Use of albuterol or a rescue inhaler two puffs with a spacer five to fifteen minutes prior to activity helps prevent exercise induced asthma symptoms.

Exercise induced asthma is typically seen two to ten minutes after heavy exercise and not at maximum intensity exercise. Pretreatment before exercise with a rescue medicine such as albuterol is recommended to prevent exercise induced asthma symptoms. If a rescue medication such as albuterol is needed more than once per day, a controller medication or long-term asthma medicine is usually added.

Warming up is important to decrease exercise induced asthma symptoms caused by cold air. The nose warms, filters, and moistens air entering the airway. Kids should learn to breathe in through their nose and out through their mouth when exercising. In addition, children should warm-up with a mask or scarf over the mouth if exercising in cold air.

Physical activity is recommended for all children to keep them healthy. Although the age old saying "use it or lose it" does not necessarily apply to children with asthma, it is important to encourage children with asthma to exercise. Weight gain is associated with worsened outcome in asthma. Children with exercise induced asthma are more likely to limit their physical activity level and be sedentary. Exercise is safe for children with asthma as long as their symptoms have been controlled with the proper medications.

Studies show low risk sports for children with exercise induced asthma include those with under ten minutes of concentrated effort such as tennis, gymnastics, golf, martial arts, fencing, track and field (sprinting 100m–400m). Higher risk for exercise induced asthma are sports requiring a high level of intensity for longer periods of time in cold or dry air, such as long-distance running, vigorous cycling, ice hockey, and ice skating. Exercise induced asthma is common in elite athletes, and those participating in endurance sports may be at higher risk, but their symptoms can usually be controlled. However, children competing in endurance exercises who are poorly controlled may experience stress, inflammation, and damage of the airways with repeated high intensity or long duration workouts.

Expert Tip

Exercise induced asthma is present in 30 to 70 percent of Olympic level athletes depending on the sport and reporting methods.

Walking or hiking is less likely to trigger asthma symptoms unless you are at higher elevations where there is less oxygen in the air. Walking or hiking in cold, dry air should be avoided. When I was growing up, swimming was thought to be a great exercise for asthmatics. However, now we know swimming may not be safe for all asthmatics. Chlorine is an airway irritant that may trigger bronchoconstriction. In addition, swimming for long periods of time with high intensity may increase the risk for an asthma attack. Low intensity or leisurely swimming is safer for most asthmatics. Yoga is an excellent exercise for children and teens with asthma. Specifically, hot yoga may lessen the loss of humidity from the airway mucosa or lining suspected to cause bronchoconstriction. Leisurely biking is also a great exercise for asthmatics. A temperate climate may decrease the risk of asthma symptoms.

An asthma attack is frightening, and most children understandably panic when they have one. As the parent, coach, or care provider, you should try to calm the child down and administer albuterol. For children, a spacer device (tube-like inhaler extension) is recommended to assist with proper deposition of the medication into the lungs. If albuterol is not available, the child should be coached to breathe in through their nose and out through their mouth. In addition, emergency services should be called to provide medical treatment.

What Happens During an Asthma Attack?

It can be frustrating for parents and kids that despite taking all medications as prescribed, an asthma exacerbation or attack can still happen. Worst of all, they are unpredictable. An asthma trigger causes a cascade of inflammatory cells in the airway leading to aggravation of persistent airway swelling and bronchoconstriction or narrowing of the airway. The asthma trigger could be any number of possible suspects such as illness, exercise, or an environmental exposure. Of course, avoiding triggers helps eliminate the risk of an asthma attack. But sometimes removing the trigger is not possible. For instance, if you are an athlete with exercise induced asthma, the activity you love the most such as running, swimming, or football may also increase the chance of asthma exacerbation. This does not mean you have to limit activity. It does mean you should be prepared.

Expert Tip

Early use of a rescue medication like albuterol is important to keep an asthma attack from worsening. Discuss with your doctor how many puffs of albuterol or your rescue medication should be taken during an asthma attack.

During an asthma attack, symptoms are dramatically worsened. When air is forced through the narrowed airway, it causes wheezing or whistling of the airway. For example, when you pucker your lips and force air through, the sound you make is a whistle. While whistling through the lips makes a high-pitched sound, wheezing can have a musical quality with a range of timbres. Taking a look at your child's chest wall is important in knowing how severe their symptoms are. Infants and children retract or use additional muscles to open the airways when they have difficulty breathing known as respiratory distress. Abdominal breathing, pulling in of the chest underneath the rib cage, pulling of muscles in-between the ribs, or a depression at the base of the neck all are retractions. Tachypnea or fast respiratory rate is a sensitive sign of respiratory distress in infants and young children. Nasal flaring or expanding of the nostrils is a sign that your child is having difficulty breathing.

Expert Tip

Most young children with asthma do not cough up or expectorate their mucus, so it may continue to block the airway. If they do cough up mucus, often it is swallowed, upsetting the stomach and causing vomiting.

For older children, an asthma attack may just be coughing, wheezing, or breathlessness without retractions. The symptoms may start slowly, or onset may be sudden. Kids often complain their chest or "heart" hurts. Most kids will want to sit down and rest. Pallor of the face or cyanosis (blueness) of the lips and tongue may happen. When the airway stops making noises and is quiet during an attack, this is ominous and indicates the airway is completely closed down. When the lungs cannot function efficiently, both the lungs and heart work harder. If the lungs are unable to deliver needed oxygen to the body, the system shuts down, and this is called respiratory failure.

Expert Tip

Asthma symptoms tend to worsen in the evening.
If your child's symptoms are concerning in the early evening, they are usually not going to be better overnight. Call the doctor or go to the urgent care or emergency department early in the evening. This will prevent a middle of the night trip to the hospital.

Time is precious during an asthma attack, and the symptoms will escalate if you do not intervene. The most important way to minimize the severity of an asthma attack is to act quickly. Use of a fast-acting rescue medication like albuterol is the first line of defense. Make sure you have clear instructions from your doctor about which medicine you should give and how much when your child has an asthma attack. If your child's symptoms are not improved with the medicine, you should call emergency services or go to the emergency department.

How Is Asthma Treated?

There are two major types of medications that treat asthma, rescue and controller medications. A rescue medication is fast-acting and works quickly to open the airway by loosening the muscle around the airway, alleviating bronchoconstriction and asthma symptoms. The effects of a rescue medication are short-lived and do not fix the underlying swelling of the airway. A long-term control medication is taken daily to decrease inflammation in the airway and resolve asthma symptoms.

Expert Tip

When reviewing asthma medications, keep in mind they usually have two names for the same medication, the generic and the brand or trade name.

Rescue Medications

Albuterol is the most common rescue medication for asthma. Albuterol is the generic name for Proair®, Ventolin®, and Proventil®. Albuterol works by bronchodilation or loosening the muscle wrapping around the airway. The onset of action is five to ten minutes, and the medication lasts for three to six hours. Albuterol may be administered by nebulization, a mist of medicine delivered by a machine, or an inhaler device. Common side effects of albuterol include fast heart rate (tachycardia) or tremors. Albuterol delivers 90mcg per puff from the inhaler. There are nebulized formulations of varying strengths.

Expert Tip

There are several manufacturers for albuterol, and the inhaler may be red, yellow, or blue. However, the pharmaceutical company can change the color of the packaging or medication. It's important you know the name of your medication and not just the color.

Levalbuterol is the generic name for Xopenex˚, a medication similar to albuterol but with a different chemical structure. Xopenex˚ also causes bronchodilation of the airway quickly in five to ten minutes and lasts for three to six hours. Common side effects of Xopenex˚ include fast heart rate (tachycardia) or tremor. Xopenex˚ delivers 45mcg of levalbuterol per puff from the inhaler. There are nebulized formulations of varying strengths.

> ### *Expert Tip*
>
> Technique is important to ensure the medication from an asthma inhaler or nebulizer actually makes it to the lungs. A spacer device is a tube that attaches to an asthma inhaler in order to effectively deliver the medication to the airway. With a nebulizer, always use a mask firmly fitted to the face. Blow by nebulization does not reliably deliver medicine.

Long-Term Control Medications

The purpose of a long-term control medication is to decrease airway inflammation, that if left unchecked leads to airway remodeling, loss of lung function, and reduced lung growth in children. The type and dose of controller medication prescribed is based upon the age of the child and the severity of the asthma symptoms. A controller medication is indicated if a child: requires albuterol more than two days per week during the past four weeks, has two or more asthma exacerbations requiring oral steroids in six months, has shortness of breath during normal activity, or has decreased lung function.

Inhaled corticosteroids (ICS) are the most effective long-term control medications available to treat mild, moderate, or severe persistent asthma. They work by inhibiting airway inflammation and blocking response to allergens at the airway lining with little systemic absorption. Kids should rinse their mouth after use of inhaled steroids to prevent thrush or a yeast infection of the mouth. Inhaled corticosteroids are not addictive. Parents are frequently concerned about side effects of inhaled steroids.

> ### *Expert Tip*
>
> Don't worry; inhaled corticosteroids will not turn your fifth grader into a rippling body builder. This class of medication is different than anabolic steroids used by some athletes to illegally enhance athletic performance.

Kids at highest risk of side effects from ICS are those taking high doses of ICS for over one year or in combination with oral steroids. The most significant side effects of inhaled corticosteroids are slowing down of growth, adrenal gland suppression, and decreased bone mineral density. Growth delay with use of ICS is usually slight and no more than about one centimeter. Use of inhaled steroids for brief periods of time typically does not impact final adult height. However, it is important that inhaled steroids are discontinued when not needed or the dose weaned, as tolerated, when asthma control is achieved. To be clear, the benefits of inhaled corticosteroids for treatment of asthma outweigh the risks. The risk of side effects is much higher with use of systemic steroids, meaning the entire body is exposed to steroids taken by oral or intravenous route.

> ### *Expert Tip*
>
> One of the goals of asthma treatment is to use the least amount of medicine possible to reduce the risk of asthma and impairment caused by the disease.

There are several inhaled steroids on the market from which to choose. Most ICS are covered by Medicaid formularies, but for private insurance, depending on the type of insurance coverage, can be expensive. Check with your doctor and pharmacist to see if there are coupons available to decrease the expense of asthma medications.

Different types of delivery systems are available for asthma inhalers. A pressurized metered dose inhaler (pMDI) contains the drug and a propellant which delivers medication to the airway. Hydrofluoroalkane (HFA) is the most common propellant used in pressurized metered dose inhalers. Correct technique when using an inhaler device is important to ensure medication from an inhaler deposits in the lungs. A spacer device assists with effective delivery of the medication to the airway in children with difficulty coordinating their breathing. Without a spacer device, medication from some inhalers will land on the back of the throat or is swallowed, never reaching the lungs. In children from birth up to three years of age, a pressurized metered dose inhaler and a dedicated spacer with a face mask is recommended. Alternatively, in a child from birth to three years of age, a nebulizer with face mask may be used. In children four to five years, a pMDI with a dedicated spacer and mouthpiece is recommended or a nebulizer with mouthpiece/face mask attachment. Dry powder inhalers (DPI) do not require a propellant and are breath activated by the child. Children as young as four years of age can generate enough flow to deliver medication from DPIs. However, some children may have difficulty coordinating their breathing with these devices. Small-particle inhaled corticosteroids use an extra-fine particle that can deposit deeper in the airways.

For children twelve months and older, the following ICS are recommended:
- Budesonide nebulizer solution (Trade Name: Pulmicort˚)
  - » Use only a jet nebulizer

For children four years and older, the following ICS are recommended:
- Fluticasone propionate (HFA/standard particle/ pMDI) (Trade Name: Flovent˚)

For children over five years of age, the following ICS are recommended:

- Budesonide (pMDI/ standard particle/extra-fine particle/ DPI)

- Fluticasone Fuorate (DPI) Not sufficiently studied in children
- Beclomethasone (HFA extra-fine particle) (Trade Name: QVAR˚)
- Flunisolide (HFA) (built-in spacer)
- Ciclesonide (pMDI/extra-fine particle/HFA)
  » Children over five only
- Triamcinolone acetonide (pMDI) (Trade Name: Azmacort®)
- Mometasone Furoate (standard particle/HFA/pMDI) (Trade Name: Asmanex˚)

Expert Tip

About 50-80 percent of the dose from the pMDI without a spacer is swallowed, never reaching the lungs.
So, spacer use with inhalers is strongly urged.

When ICS do not control asthma symptoms, a different type of asthma medication is needed. Combination ICS medications are inhaled corticosteroids with a long-acting rescue medication called a long-acting beta$_2$ agonist (LABA). The benefit of these medications is a reduced need for recurrent use of short-acting rescue medications like albuterol.

For children over five years of age, following combined medication is recommended:

- Fluticasone/Salmeterol (DPI/pMDI) (Trade Name: Advair˚)

For children twelve years of age and older. the following combined medications are recommended:

- Mometasone/Formoterol pMDI (Trade Name: Dulera˚)
- Budesonide/Formoterol pMDI (Trade Name: Symbicort˚)

<u>Antileukotrienes/leukotriene modifiers</u> are medications that block leukotrienes, a substance causing mucus production, bronchoconstriction, and inflammation. This class of medication is less effective than inhaled corticosteroids but helpful as an accompanying therapy when used with inhaled corticosteroids. Some children respond well to leukotriene modifiers/antileukotrienes alone. However, there is no way to predict or be certain a child will benefit from leukotriene modifiers.

For children twelve months and older, the following leukotriene modifiers are available:

- Montelukast (Trade Name: Singulair˚)
  - » Side effect- neuropsychiatric events including behavior and mood-related changes including suicidal thoughts or actions

For children five years and older, the following leukotriene modifiers are available:

- Zafirlukast (Trade Name: Accolate®)
  - » Rarely used

Expert Tip

Asthma medications only work if you take them. Children must take 80 percent of their medication doses for the medicine to be effective. If you are prescribed a twice daily medication, you need to take eleven of fourteen doses per week.

Long-acting muscarinic antagonists (LAMAs) are medications used in children with severe asthma that is difficult to manage. These medications block certain chemicals in the body, causing loosening of airway muscle and a decrease in production of secretions. They are not fast-acting so are not rescue medications, but are used for improved control of asthma.

For children six years and older, the following LAMA is available.

- Tiotropium (DPI) (Trade Name: Spiriva® Respimat®)

Expert Tip

If your child takes oral steroids or steroids by mouth (prednisolone or prednisone) repeatedly, they are at higher risk for side effects when compared to using low dose inhaled steroids routinely.

<u>Oral steroids</u> are used in children with moderate to severe persistent asthma with exacerbation of their symptoms. They have an onset of action of two hours and are not fast-acting. Oral steroids work by decreasing airway swelling and secretions. Treatment with oral steroids usually lasts two to five days. Side effects of these medications include oral steroid dependency, weight gain, increased risk for diabetes, high blood pressure, behavioral changes, decreased growth, decreased bone mineral density, adrenal insufficiency, and headache. Using oral steroids intermittently is higher risk than using inhaled steroids daily.

For children of all ages, the following oral steroid are available:

- Methylprednisolone
- Prednisolone
- Prednisone
- Dexamethasone
    - » Frequently used in the emergency department

<u>Biologic agents</u> or immunomodulators are medications targeting specific inflammatory pathways associated with asthma. Biologic drugs are produced by living cells through processes that mimic the natural biological parts of our body like antibodies. These are injectable medications approved for use in children with difficult to treat asthma, not improved with traditional asthma medications. Children requiring two or more bursts of oral steroids for greater than three days or at least one hospitalization in the previous year also qualify for biologic medications. Each biologic medication has a different mechanism of action and requires specific lab testing to determine if a child with severe persistent asthma or uncontrolled asthma is eligible. There is a risk of anaphylaxis or severe allergic reaction with all of these medications. Epinephrine is typically prescribed for patients using biologic agents due to the risk of anaphylaxis.

For children six years and older, the following biologic medications are available:

- Omalizumab (Trade Name: Xolair*)
  - » Injection every two to four weeks
- Mepolizumab (Trade Name: Nucala*)
  - » Injection every four weeks

For children twelve years and older, the following biologic medications are available:
- Benralizumab (Trade Name: Fasenra*)

- » Injection every four weeks for the first three doses, then eight weeks
- » Can be given at home

- Dupilumab (Trade Name: Dupixent˚)
  - » Injection every two weeks
  - » Can be given at home

Omalizumab (Xolair˚) is the biologic agent on the market for the longest and is an anti-IgE immunoglobulin. It was first approved for use in 2003. Omalizumab binds to free IgE, preventing IgE from reaching its receptor (place of action) thereby reducing asthma symptoms. With this medication, children have achieved reduced use of inhaled steroids, oral steroids, and asthma exacerbations. Patients six years of age and older with an elevated IgE level and allergies are eligible for Xolair˚.

Mepolizumab (Nucala˚) binds to an inflammatory substance in the body and prevents eosinophil induced asthma response. Patients six years of age and over with increased eosinophils qualify for Nucala˚. There is improvement in asthma control and a reduction of asthma exacerbations with Nucala˚.

Benralizumab (Fasenra˚) reduces sputum and blood eosinophils and decreases asthma exacerbation rates. The exact mechanism of action or way it works is not fully understood. It is approved for children twelve years and older and can be administered at home.

Dupilimab (Dupixent˚) works by blocking inflammatory particles in the body that lead to asthma response. It reduces asthma exacerbation rates and severe eczema. Dupixent˚ can be administered at home, which is a major advantage for most families.

Which Asthma Medications Should My Child Take?

A stepwise approach is used to build an asthma plan. Your doctor will determine which medication and what dose are appropriate. The following provides case studies that are examples of children with asthma symptoms and how they should be treated. An asthma treatment regimen for a child is based upon their asthma severity classification and age. Keep in mind, your child's plan may be very different depending on their clinical history. (***The following *is not* a treatment recommendation for your child but simply a general guide which should be adjusted by your child's doctor.)

Case Study 1:

Alice is a five-year-old girl who recently started kindergarten. She wheezes when she is sick and the temperature changes. Fortunately, she does not have symptoms very often. Her doctor has never prescribed an oral steroid. She has never been to the emergency department for her symptoms.

Alice is classified as having intermittent asthma. She does not need a daily medication for asthma.

Intermittent Asthma

Treatment for All Ages:

Rescue Medication: Albuterol two puffs with a spacer every four hours as needed for cough or wheezing

Control Medication: None

Case Study 2:

Chase is eight years old, and she loves to swim and play outside. During the last six months, her mother notices she coughs three to four days per week even when she is not playing. She has a runny nose when she plays outside. Her pediatrician started an antihistamine for allergies, and she uses albuterol when she coughs. She wakes up two nights per month with shortness of breath and difficulty breathing. She needed two courses of prednisone this year for persistent cough after a cold and the flu. She has never taken a daily inhaled medication for her respiratory symptoms. Chase has mild persistent asthma and needs daily medications for asthma.

Mild Persistent Asthma

Treatment for All Ages:

Rescue Medication: Albuterol two puffs with a spacer every four hours as needed for cough or wheezing

Control Medication: Flovent® 44mcg two puffs twice daily with a spacer device (rinse mouth after use) + montelukast

---

Expert Tip

Poorly controlled asthma can slow growth.

Case Study 3:

Brooke is four years old, and Amanda is six years old. They are sisters who look alike and do everything together. Their parents smoke and have asthma. Brooke and Amanda both have asthma symptoms every day including cough and shortness of breath. Brooke awakens overnight for difficulty breathing three to four times per month, and Amanda awakens overnight one time per week. They use albuterol daily for their cough. Both sisters have been to the emergency department three times this year for asthma exacerbation with oral steroids prescribed. Currently, they are both using Flovent® 44mcg, two puffs twice a day without a spacer device.

Both Brooke and Amanda are classified as having Moderate Persistent Asthma. They both would benefit from using a stronger daily inhaled steroid and spacer device to ensure better deposition in the airway. Brook and Amanda should be increased to Flovent® 110mcg, one puff with a spacer device twice daily for improved control of their asthma. This plan keeps things easy for their parents, as both girls are on the same medication. However, Amanda can also be treated with a combination (ICS/LABA) like Advair® and montelukast (antileukotriene) to improve asthma symptoms because she is six. Their parents should be urged to quit smoking and avoid smoking in the house and car.

Moderate Persistent Asthma

Children birth to four years:

Rescue Medication: Albuterol two puffs with a spacer every four hours as needed for cough or wheezing

Control Medication: Flovent® 110mcg, one puff twice daily with a spacer device (rinse mouth after use)

Children five to 11 years:

Rescue Medication: Albuterol two puffs with a spacer every four hours as needed for cough or wheezing

Control Medication: Advair® 45/21mcg, one inhalation twice daily with a spacer device (rinse mouth after use) + montelukast

OR Flovent® 110mcg, one puff twice daily with a spacer device (rinse mouth after use)

Children twelve or older

Rescue Medication: Albuterol two puffs with a spacer every four hours as needed for cough or wheezing

Control Medication: Advair® 115/21mcg, one inhalation twice daily with a spacer device (rinse mouth after use) OR

Flovent ® 110mcg, two puffs twice daily with a spacer device (rinse mouth after use)

Case Study 4:

Mathew is a sixteen-year-old male who played football and ran track last year. During this school year, he attends virtual school and has not been as active. He has gained some weight. Mathew enjoys playing video games and usually stays up late. He eats spicy chips late at night which cause heartburn and cough. He used to take Flovent 110mcg, two puffs twice a day but stopped this when he started virtual school. Mathew had COVID-19 about six weeks ago and has developed a persistent dry cough during the day and overnight. He is using albuterol two to three times per day for his cough. This year he needed oral steroids twice for asthma exacerbations. He used to vape three to four times per week but now does it only once per week.

The frequency of Mathew's symptoms make him a severe persistent asthmatic. However, he has other risk factors for conditions that could worsen asthma, like reflux. Mathew's story illustrates how asthma symptoms may be worsened by weight gain, respiratory illness, smoking/vaping, and noncompliance with medications. Mathew would benefit from asthma education and regular use of a combination medication (ICS/LABA) like Advair®, Symbicort®, or Dulera® in addition to montelukast (antileukotriene). It would be a good idea to treat his reflux because it may worsen his asthma. He should stop smoking/vaping. He needs a chest x-ray and should be referred to a pediatric pulmonologist.

Severe Persistent Asthma

<u>Children birth to four years</u>

Rescue Medication: Albuterol, two puffs with a spacer every four hours as needed for cough or wheezing

Control Medication: Flovent® 110mcg, one puff twice daily with a spacer device (rinse mouth after use) + montelukast

<u>Children five to eleven years</u>

Rescue Medication: Albuterol two puffs with a spacer every four hours as needed for cough or wheezing

Control Medication: Advair ® 115/21mcg, one inhalation twice daily with a spacer device (rinse mouth after use) OR Flovent ® 110mcg, one puff twice daily with a spacer device (rinse mouth after use) +montelukast

<u>Children twelve or older </u>

Rescue Medication: Albuterol two puffs with a spacer every four hours as needed for cough or wheezing

Control Medication: Advair® 115/21mcg, two inhalations twice daily with a spacer device (rinse mouth after use) + montelukast OR Flovent® 220mcg, two puffs twice daily with a spacer device (rinse mouth after use) + montelukast

Is My Child's Asthma Controlled?

Controlling asthma is important to decrease the risk of asthma exacerbations, prevent ED visits or hospitalizations, stop loss of lung function, and avoid reduced lung growth. To determine if your child's asthma is controlled, you must assess the frequency of symptoms, use of a rescue medication, and lung function. If your child has well-controlled asthma, they should have normal lung function, no interference with normal activity, and follow the rule of twos:

- Asthma symptoms no more than two times per week
- Nighttime awakenings no more than two times per month (children eleven years of age and younger cough no more than one time per month)
- Needs albuterol no more than two days per week (excluding exercise)
- Less than two asthma exacerbations per year requiring oral steroids

What Is My Asthma Strategy?

Controlling asthma requires a strategy, dedicated care team, and commitment to the plan. From my standpoint, there are five essential steps to successful management of asthma. I call it DRIVE.

D-*Detail*

R-*Ready for Action*

I- *Investment*

V-*Verification*

E-*Exit Plan*

This is a philosophy derived from years of experience, both having asthma personally and treating kids with asthma. Following the steps of this strategy empowers you to be an excellent partner with your doctor. Let's explore further what DRIVE means as you embark on this journey to diagnose and treat asthma symptoms.

Detail

Kids are dependent on parents or caregivers to be their health advocate and representative. The information parents or caregivers provide doctors called the medical history is critical to ensuring the correct diagnosis is made. Your power as a parent or caregiver is knowing your child better than anyone. When your doctor asks you about how and when respiratory symptoms happen, it is important you provide detailed information and think broadly about your child's medical history. Were they premature, or did they have episodes of viral bronchiolitis as an infant or toddler? Did he or she have pneumonia or frequent respiratory illness from a certain age? If you have a hard time remembering these facts because it was a long time ago or you have several kids, enlist the help of a grandparent, partner, or spouse to jog your memory in preparation for your office visit. Write down the information you want to tell your doctor before the visit, so you do not forget important information. Also, make sure you ask questions about symptoms your child has. Most doctors will give you their working diagnosis that may include other conditions besides asthma. Remember to give specific information about what medications your child has already taken and include any alternative therapy or over-the-counter medications you have tried. Don't forget to tell your doctor about any surgeries and medication allergies or reactions. Remind your doctor if your child had any testing such as chest x-rays or allergy skin tests. Make sure you have copies of the study results to give to your doctor at the time of the visit. Review if your child has any other diagnoses or sees a specialist for any conditions. Check with relatives about family history of asthma and allergies. A detail-oriented approach ensures all pertinent information about your child is included for consideration when a diagnosis of asthma is contemplated.

Ready for Action

When your child receives a diagnosis of asthma, you must be ready for action. Symptoms will only improve if you follow the plan provided by your doctor and give the medication to your child. Asthma symptoms can be unpredictable and rapidly worsen if you encounter a trigger. Your child should have their rescue medication, for most an albuterol inhaler with a spacer, available for use at all times. Children who have exercise induced asthma may need to take albuterol two puffs with a spacer device five to fifteen minutes prior to activity, called albuterol premedication. Make sure you request letters from your doctor to authorize emergency use of albuterol for a school or day care. Educate anyone who provides care for your child (coach, teacher, grandparent) about possible asthma symptoms and how to treat them. Make sure when your child has an asthma attack you do not panic. Remember, you have a plan, and staying calm helps you follow the doctor's instructions. Organization matters when it comes to treating asthma successfully. If you are prepared, you will always be ready for action when asthma symptoms happen unexpectedly.

Investment

Patience is a virtue with asthma care. Improvement happens slowly, but worsened symptoms are quickly noticeable. Expect to take new asthma medications for at least two to three months to determine if there are clear benefits. Young children especially have frequent viral illnesses that worsen respiratory status. It is hard to know for sure if asthma medications are ineffective or whether illness has sabotaged your medicine's positive effect. If you abandon your asthma plan too quickly, you will never know if it was going to work. Your child's care team includes not only your doctors but teachers, coaches, grandparents, family, and friends. Make sure everyone is aware of your child's diagnosis of asthma and invested in making your plan successful. Invite your family and friends to help you assess how respiratory symptoms change over time. Keeping an asthma diary over two to four weeks helps you remember what happened after starting the medication. An asthma diary can be created on a cell phone or in a journal. You should record what time your child took medications and how often you forgot. Most patients forget to give at least one to two doses per week. If you have forgotten to give most doses of the medication or the child takes it sporadically, a true assessment of how medications work is not possible. If you don't give medications as prescribed, you should not expect a change in your child's symptoms. Kids love stickers and prizes. Make an asthma calendar and add stickers when your child successfully takes their asthma medications each day. Keep the calendar visible and encourage them to take ownership of the medication. For older kids, figure out how you can incentivize taking medications with rewards your child or teen will enjoy. Young children and 'tweens need supervision when taking daily medications and sometimes, teenagers too. For infant and toddlers, taking asthma medications does not have to be a battle. Getting them to tolerate a face mask with a spacer device or the nebulizer mask can be challenging. Mask desensitization involves removing fear of mask use by playing with it apart from use with the medication and making the medicine use part of a game. With time, young children often will accept the mask and sit through their treatments. The time and effort you invest in making your asthma plan successful is worth the reward of improved asthma symptoms.

Verification

Once a diagnosis of asthma is given, symptoms must be reassessed to determine if asthma is controlled. This requires a return visit to your doctor to verify improvement in symptoms. If a child's symptoms are unchanged, perhaps stronger medication is needed, or there are additional co-morbidities (other conditions) making asthma symptoms worse, like reflux. There are some children who do not have asthma. Instead, they may have a separate diagnosis mimicking asthma. If a diagnosis of asthma is in doubt due to poor response to asthma treatment, referral to a pediatric pulmonologist or lung specialist for kids may be needed. If asthma symptoms are improved, medications are usually continued.

Expert Tip

Children with asthma do not become addicted to asthma medications. Stopping an asthma medication abruptly increases the risk for asthma symptoms returning.

Exit Plan

When your child's asthma symptoms are controlled and you have been giving medications routinely for three months, it is time to assess if you can wean medications. By weaning, I mean decreasing the dose to determine if less medication will still effectively control symptoms. Some parents and kids are fearful of this process because they are so traumatized by the severity of illness experienced before the winning combination of medications were found. Others are elated to know less medication is possible. The beauty of caring for kids is they grow, change, and develop each month. Asthma symptoms are often seasonal, waxing and waning depending on multiple variables. A care plan working well for a child is always reassuring; however, there is risk involved with continuing asthma medications long-term. How and when to stop medication is specific to your child's symptom severity and pattern. Make sure you follow up regularly with your doctor, so they can assess symptoms over time and provide you with a specific plan of how and when to wean asthma medications. If you want to stop your child's asthma medications, check with your doctor first. It is best to stop just one medication at a time and to wait at least two weeks between stopping medications. Then if symptoms worsen, you know which medication your child really needs.

Now that you understand the asthma success strategy DRIVE, you are ready for your asthma road map called an Asthma Action Plan. All patients with asthma should have an Asthma Action Plan provided by their doctor. It clearly lists what medications should be taken and how much medication should be administered. The following Asthma Action Plan is an example of what your doctor may give you. Make sure you keep the Asthma Action Plan your doctor gives you with your child's medications.

ASTHMA ACTION PLAN

			HOW MUCH	HOW OFTEN
	GREEN MEANS GO! ASTHMA SYMPTOMS ARE GOOD	CONTROLLER MEDICINE (Take This Everyday) WITH EXERCISE TAKE THIS MEDICINE		
	YELLOW MEANS CAUTION! ADD QUICK RELIEF MEDICATION	RESCUE MEDICINE	HOW MUCH	HOW OFTEN
	RED MEANS DANGER! GET HELP FROM DOCTOR	RESCUE MEDICINE CALL THE DOCTOR PHONE:	HOW MUCH	HOW OFTEN

When Do I Go to the Emergency Department?

If your child has difficulty breathing and does not respond to a rescue medication like albuterol at home, they should be taken to the emergency department (ED), urgent care, or emergency medical services (911) should be called. When you arrive at the ED, if your child is in respiratory distress, they should be assessed immediately to determine if they need oxygen. This is done with a pulse oximeter, a device measuring the oxygen level in the blood through a probe placed on the fingertip or toe. Normal oxygen levels are 92 percent or higher via pulse oximetry. If oxygen levels are low, supplemental oxygen should be administered. In the ED, asthma exacerbations are treated with continuous albuterol and other rescue medications. Your child will be placed on a cardiac and respiratory monitor to observe vital signs while medications are administered.

Expert Tip

Albuterol should not be administered at home closer together than every four hours. Albuterol can cause fast heart rate (tachycardia) or other changes causing arrhythmia or abnormal heart rhythm if given in high doses.

Hospitals have varying protocols for which medications are used during an asthma exacerbation. Oral steroids (dexamethasone, prednisone) are usually given prior to discharge and prescribed for home. Keep in mind when you leave the ED, your child is still at risk for worsened asthma symptoms. If environmental risk factors at home such as dust, smoke exposure, or mold are triggers for your child's asthma, returning home may cause the symptoms to recur. It is important to follow up with your pediatrician within twenty-four hours of an ED visit to determine if additional testing or medications are needed.

My Child Is Hospitalized with Asthma – What Should I Do?

An admission to the hospital for an asthma exacerbation is worrisome and scary for parents and for children. Contact your pediatrician immediately to make them aware of your child's hospitalization for asthma. Verify with the inpatient doctors if your child had a chest x-ray and ask if they have pneumonia or other signs of infection. Review any lab studies completed and ask if your child has been tested for respiratory viruses. Discuss with the hospital respiratory therapist what technique they used to administer asthma medications. If your child is not improving after twenty-four hours, ask for a detailed explanation of the medical plan. Do not be afraid to ask for a hospital consultation from the pediatric pulmonologist or to have your pediatrician discuss your child's care with the inpatient team. Make sure you understand what medications are being given in the hospital and which medications you should continue at home. You are your child's advocate and voice. Feel empowered to speak up and ensure your child receives the best care possible. Follow up with your pediatrician twenty-four hours after a hospitalization and determine if additional testing for asthma is needed or different medications should be prescribed.

Does My Child Need a Lung Specialist or Pediatric Pulmonologist?

If asthma medications are not working to resolve your child's symptoms or your child has been hospitalized for asthma, you should be seen by a lung specialist to figure out why. All coughing and wheezing are not caused by asthma. Maybe your child does not have asthma, or perhaps the optimal asthma plan has not been created. A lung specialist for kids or pediatric pulmonologist can provide the next steps for evaluation. If needed, they can complete additional blood testing for infections or immunodeficiency, lung function testing (spirometry), and a flexible bronchoscopy, or insertion of a bendable tube with a camera in the airway to directly visualize airway passages while obtaining lung fluid for analysis.

Pediatric pulmonologists are trained with the skills of a doctor detective to determine why your child is still sick. A detailed history of symptom onset, triggers, and exacerbating and alleviating factors is critical. When you visit with the pulmonologist come prepared to answer lots of questions. Make sure you have written down your concerns and take notes during the visit. It is helpful to record the concerning event and show the video at the visit.

Keep reading to review the list of conditions that mimic asthma or co-exist with asthma and are commonly treated by pediatric pulmonologists. Understanding what disorders cause coughing or wheezing but are not asthma helps you point your doctor toward the correct diagnosis. Understanding the disorders reviewed below will help you determine if your child has asthma or one of the other conditions that may be mistaken for asthma. Keep in mind, if some of these conditions are present in addition to asthma, it makes a diagnosis of asthma more complex.

Viral Bronchiolitis

In children less than two years of age, viral illness causing swelling of the small airway or bronchioles is the most frequent cause of wheezing. Other symptoms of viral bronchiolitis include chest congestion, runny nose, fever, and for more severe cases may include retractions, fast respiratory rate (tachypnea), apnea, or development of respiratory distress. Rhinovirus, the common cold, and respiratory syncytial virus (RSV) often are the source of infection. Treatment is supportive care with fluids and fever reducers (acetaminophen). Unfortunately, studies show albuterol does not work to speed recovery from bronchiolitis. However, if a child has asthma and bronchiolitis or severe bronchiolitis, there are benefits to giving a trial of albuterol. Steroids are not used routinely in the treatment of a first-time case of bronchiolitis. If a child has recurrent bronchiolitis with hospitalization, they are at higher risk for having asthma and may benefit from starting asthma medications including steroids.

Aspiration

Aspiration is inhalation of foreign material into the airway. Children may aspirate due to anatomic (structural) abnormalities, neurological concerns, or developmental issues. Aspiration may originate from the mouth while swallowing or from below if stomach contents are refluxed. There is no way for the lung to completely break down food particles. Aspiration causes irritation of the airway leading to infection or lung injury. Kids who aspirate typically cough or gag while eating or drinking. Sometimes aspiration is silent, and the child does not reveal their swallow dysfunction. Diagnosis of aspiration is commonly completed by a videofluoroscopic swallow study or modified barium swallow (MBS) with a speech therapist. During a swallow study or MBS, different consistencies of barium, a substance visible during an x-ray, are fed to a child to determine if food is entering the airway. Direct visualization of the airway with surgical laryngoscopy (camera view of larynx) or flexible bronchoscopy (bendable camera view of airway) may be needed.

Chronic Lung Disease of Prematurity

Children born prematurely with an oxygen requirement for twenty-eight days after birth are classified as having chronic lung disease (CLD) or bronchopulmonary dysplasia. They are at increased risk for respiratory infections, specifically RSV, and hospitalization for respiratory symptoms in the first year of life. Episodes of wheezing are common in preemies with CLD, and they may have recurrent bronchiolitis. Most infants with CLD go on to develop asthma-like symptoms when they are older and often are diagnosed with asthma. They may respond to use of inhaled corticosteroids but typically not as efficiently as children with asthma. Some patients with CLD have worsened symptoms with albuterol due to airway floppiness or malacia. When albuterol causes bronchodilation, it loosens the muscle around the airway which also gives the airway structure. Some children with CLD may respond better to ipratropium bromide (Trade Name: Atrovent*) to open the airway instead of albuterol due to airway malacia.

Foreign Body

Remember that toy, grape, hot dog, or peanut your toddler choked on a few weeks ago? That could be the cause of your child's persistent cough unresolved with asthma medications. A foreign body (FB) is an object in the airway that should not be present. Young children explore through their mouths, and about 75 percent of children with foreign body aspiration are one to three years of age. Most foreign bodies end up in the right lung because of the wider angle of the right bronchus. If complete airway obstruction is present, a child will not be able to speak or breathe. Back blows should be given to infants, and the Heimlich maneuver should be used in older children to dislodge the obstruction. Definitive diagnosis of a foreign body involves additional imaging of the chest with a chest x-ray or chest computed tomography (CT), a three- dimensional view of the chest. A flexible bronchoscopy completed by the pediatric pulmonologist can directly visualize the foreign body, and a rigid bronchoscopy (non-bendable camera in airway) can be completed to safely remove the object.

Vocal Cord Dysfunction

The vocal cords are housed in the larynx or voice box. When vocal cords close abnormally, they can cause neck or chest tightness, hoarseness, and difficulty breathing. A wheezing sound may be produced that mimics asthma. Kids with vocal cord dysfunction (VCD) usually have more difficulty inhaling. Asthma medications are not helpful because the lower airway is not involved. Triggers for VCD may be reflux, allergic rhinitis with post-nasal drip, stress, or anxiety. Treatment may include referral to speech therapy for breathing exercises, relaxation techniques, biofeedback, allergy medications, and ipratropium bromide (Trade Name: Atrovent˚). VCD may co-exist with asthma. If a child has both diagnoses, albuterol should also be considered for treatment.

Laryngomalacia

The larynx is a structure in the upper airway housing the vocal cords. When the larynx is floppy (malacia) the tissues above the vocal cords fall into the airway with inhalation creating stridor, a high-pitched squeaky sound made while breathing. Laryngomalacia or a floppy larynx is the most common cause of noisy breathing in infants. Usually, the noisiness is worse when infants are on their back and moving around, improving when they are still or on their abdomen. Infants with mild laryngomalacia breathe and feed well with resolution of symptoms by twelve to eighteen months. With moderate to severe laryngomalacia infants have difficulty feeding, spit up, apnea (stop breathing), and poor weight gain sometimes necessitating surgical intervention by an otolaryngologist or ear, nose, and throat (ENT) doctor.

Croup

A barking cough is classic for croup, an infection of the larynx or voice box. Children with croup also may have fever, hoarseness, or stridor, a squeaky sound while breathing. Croup is caused by viral illness and is most common in children age six months to three years of age. Parainfluenza 1 virus is the most frequent cause of croup during the fall and winter months. Children with severe symptoms of croup may drool, have difficulty swallowing, persistent stridor, and difficulty breathing. They should be seen in the emergency department. If your child has recurrent croup, they should also be referred to the ENT to rule out structural airway abnormality and have a flexible bronchoscopy.

Vascular Ring

Vascular rings happen in the fourth week of fetal development and are caused by abnormal branching of the aorta, the major blood vessel leaving the heart. A vascular ring encircles the trachea and esophagus, causing compression as an infant grows. Symptoms of a vascular ring include cough, wheezing, stridor, respiratory illness, difficulty breathing, problems swallowing, and vomiting if the esophagus is compressed. Diagnosis usually requires imaging of the heart with an echocardiogram (ultrasound of heart) and three-dimensional image of the heart with CT or magnetic resonance angiography. A pediatric pulmonologist may complete a flexible bronchoscopy for direct visualization of the airway with a camera to determine if there is anatomic (structural) compression of the trachea. Vascular rings are surgically repaired, correcting the airway compression and alleviating symptoms.

Reflux

Reflux is a condition where food passes from the stomach back to the esophagus. All infants reflux and typically the frequency decreases as infants grow, with resolution by one year of age. Reflux as an infant is associated with the development of reflux later in childhood. As many as 40 percent of children with reflux may present with respiratory symptoms only such as chest pain, wheezing, dry cough, and chest tightness. Small amounts of acid from the stomach aspirated into the lung causes bronchoconstriction. Reflux is a trigger for asthma but also can mimic asthma because reflux tends to worsen at night as does asthma. Diagnosis is completed with identification of clinical symptoms, upper gastrointestinal tract radiography (Upper GI), or endoscopy, insertion of a tube in the gastrointestinal system. A trial of anti-reflux medications is recommended if reflux independently or in conjunction with asthma is suspected.

Immunodeficiency

Recurrent infections may be a sign of immune system dysfunction. Children may have decreased numbers or functionality of immune cells. There are four major classes of immunoglobulins or components of the immune system, Immunoglobulin G (IgG), Immunoglobulin A (IgA), Immunoglobulin M (IgM), and Immunoglobulin E (IgE). Each immunoglobulin has a specific responsibility in the body. IgA is found in the respiratory and gastrointestinal tract. Selective IgA deficiency is the most common immunodeficiency and is associated with more frequent respiratory illness, allergies, and severe asthma. Children with suspected immunodeficiency should also be tested for antibody response to their vaccines. Immunodeficiency should be ruled out in any child with recurrent respiratory infections or difficult-to-control asthma.

Cystic Fibrosis

Cystic fibrosis (CF) is an inherited condition causing thick mucus, recurrent respiratory infection, and dysfunction of the gastrointestinal system causing poor absorption of nutrients. CF is diagnosed through a sweat test and genetic testing. During a sweat test, kids are painlessly stimulated to sweat, and the amount of chloride in the sweat is measured. Children with CF have an abnormal balance of the salt in their secretions and a saltier sweat. There is no cure for CF, but medications are available that improve the outcome of the disease. Children with a chronic cough unimproved with asthma medications should be tested for CF.

Primary Ciliary Dyskinesia

Primary ciliary dyskinesia (PCD) is an inherited disorder causing recurrent respiratory infections, sinusitis, ear infection, and sometimes abnormal positioning of the organs. It is caused by a defect in the cilia, hairs in the airway that work together to move mucus and secretions up and out of the tracheobronchial tree. PCD is diagnosed with a biopsy of the trachea or windpipe, and examination of the microscopic structure of the cilia. There is no cure for PCD, and patients are treated with respiratory medications to clear the airway, mucus thinners, and antibiotics.

Cough Variant Asthma

Cough may be the only presenting symptom for asthma. This can confuse parents and doctors who typically associate wheezing with asthma. Cough variant asthma is more likely in young children. It is treated the same way as asthma presenting with the typical symptoms. Some parents think my child has a little cough, no big deal. Any persistent cough should be evaluated and may be a sign the airway is irritated, inflamed, or infected.

Pertussis

This bacterial infection known as "whooping cough" causes a prolonged cough sometimes referred to as, the 100-day cough. Children often have clusters of coughing called a paroxysmal cough that may end with vomiting. Children are vaccinated for pertussis; however, if a child has a vaccine delay or is an infant with incomplete vaccinations, they are higher risk for this infection. Diagnosis can be made with a nasal swab and lab testing. Pertussis can be treated with azithromycin, an antibiotic, and early treatment helps to decrease the severity of the cough.

Protracted Bacterial Bronchitis

Protracted bacterial bronchitis is a lung infection caused by bacteria commonly associated with ear infections in kids. Young children with this illness have a frequent cough but typically do not expectorate or cough up sputum. Diagnosis requires a flexible bronchoscopy or insertion of a camera into the airway to obtain infected lung fluid. Treatment with an antibiotic for fourteen to twenty-one days usually resolves respiratory symptoms.

Habit Cough

Kids with a habit cough have a frequent, harsh, dry cough present during the day that is completely resolved while sleeping. The cough is not improved with asthma medications, antibiotics, or home remedies. Often kids with this repetitive symptom are high achievers in school. Evaluation by a psychologist or behavioral pediatrician may be helpful for behavioral modification recommendations to resolve the cough. Habit cough is a diagnosis of exclusion, meaning all other possible causes of a cough must be ruled out before diagnosing a child with habit cough.

Does Vaping Worsen Asthma?

Vaping or smoking electronic cigarettes is dangerous for children and has emerged as a major health crisis. Over three million high school students are active vapers, but many tried vaping first in middle school. Parents, if you have not asked your 'tween or teen if they are vaping, you should. If your child vapes, have a conversation with them about why they vape. The teens I care for who vape do it to fit in or because they are bored or anxious. Many teens who vape for several months admit it does not make them feel good, but they feel like they cannot stop. If your child vapes, they may need professional help to quit vaping. Letting them know it is wrong and may cause permanent lung damage is not enough. Kids are more concerned with immediate consequences than long-term effects.

Expert Tip

Almost two-thirds of kids and young adults age fifteen to twenty-four years do not know JUUL contains nicotine.

Vaping can also be called JUULing, juicing, or dabbing (involves marijuana). Electronic cigarettes or E-cigarettes are battery powered devices with a heating element burning a liquid producing an aerosol. JUUL is a popular brand shaped like a USB flash drive. JUUL pods contain as much nicotine as a pack of twenty cigarettes. Nicotine is highly addictive and can harm the adolescent brain which continues to develop into the mid-twenties. Using nicotine as a teenager can hurt parts of the brain important for control of attention, mood, impulse control, and learning. Using nicotine may also increase the risk of future drug addiction.

To effectively deliver nicotine solvents like propylene glycol and vegetable glycerin, FDA-approved food additives are used. These products are not safe to be inhaled. The ultrafine particles inhaled into the lungs are toxic and contain cancer-causing particles.

Expert Tip

Quitting vaping is critical to decrease asthma severity. Vaping is not safer than smoking and has considerable health risks including permanent lung damage.

E-cigarette or vaping product associated lung injury (EVALI) was declared an outbreak in August of 2019 when several cases of lung damage caused by vaping and vaping related complications leading to death were reported. The exact composition of many vaping products is unknown, but analysis of lung fluid from children shows marijuana and vitamin E acetate found in vape liquid have a stronger association with lung injury than nicotine.

There is evidence that vaping impairs viral response and bacterial clearance in the lungs. While in the midst of a global pandemic with COVID-19, this makes vaping even more dangerous. Studies have shown that young people who vape are at increased risk for contracting and spreading COVID-19 which is spread by aerosolized particles.

Children who vape and have developed increased cough, respiratory distress, or worsened asthma symptoms should have a chest CT or three-dimensional x-ray image of the lungs to evaluate them for lung damage. In addition, they should be seen by a pediatric pulmonologist and may benefit from having a flexible bronchoscopy.

Can I Use Natural and Alternative Remedies for Asthma?

In my patients, there is a growing interest in integrated care which is a blend of conventional biomedical approaches with safe and effective alternative or complementary medicine. We know asthma is a complex disease affected by environmental and genetic factors, as well as an altered immune system in early life. However, the full mechanism of asthma as a disease process is still unknown. The pharmaceuticals currently available to treat asthma have been well studied and their benefits proven. However, all medications have risks, and none is perfect. Many parents are completely anti-steroid and do not want to give their child daily medications.

Expert Tip

Most of the natural remedies available have not been FDA approved or tested specifically for safety in children.

A large study completed in 2004 suggested use of some vitamin supplements early on may increase the risk for asthma and food allergies in specific children. The American Academy of Pediatrics does not recommend over-the counter medications or natural remedies to treat asthma. However, despite all of this data refuting the benefit of natural remedies for asthma, many children with asthma are taking natural remedies. It is important to know what is available and safe if you would like a more natural approach to asthma management.

Vitamin D is a sunlight activated vitamin playing an important role in lung health and preventing atopy. Maternal vitamin D supplementation shows prevention of asthma and recurrent wheezing in children up to three years of age. It is important for children to get ten to thirty minutes of midday sunlight several days per week to maintain vitamin D levels. People of color with darker skin tones may need longer amounts of sunlight to activate vitamin D. Checking vitamin D levels with a blood test determines if a child needs supplementation. The correct dose needed should be discussed with your doctor. Dietary sources of vitamin D are oily fish (salmon, cod liver oil), fortified foods (milk, orange juice,) and green leafy vegetables.

Vitamin E protects against pollution damage which can trigger asthma. Vitamin E is an antioxidant, a substance that slows free radicals or unstable molecules the body produces in response to environmental stress. Dietary sources of vitamin E include almonds, peanuts, sunflower seeds, peanuts, collard greens, and spinach.

Omega-3 fatty acids are healthy oils in fish that when consumed in pregnancy can reduce asthma in children ages three to five years as shown in some studies. There may also be an association between intake of omega-3 fatty acids and decreased asthma severity in inner city children with asthma.

Garlic and ginger have anti-inflammatory effects, but there is no conclusive evidence that they improve asthma.

A Chinese herb called Ding-Chuang-Tang (DTC) anecdotally decreases inflammation and relieves bronchospasm. However, there are no conclusive studies to support this. Some herbs used to treat asthma may have dangerous side effects when interacting with other medicine. For example, licorice root is used to soothe the lungs of asthmatics but can cause increased blood pressure.

A plant-based diet or the Mediterranean diet comprised of fruits, vegetables, whole grains, nuts, seeds, and healthy fats like olive oil is associated with reduced body mass index (BMI). Elevated BMI and being overweight is an increased risk factor for asthma.

Caffeine is a mild bronchodilator and improves lung function modestly for up to four hours after use.

Mind-body medicine may be used for the treatment of pediatric asthma. Popular practices are relaxation and breathing exercises. Yoga assists with stress reduction. Biofeedback is a technique training children to control their body by using information about the body's functions recorded through devices. Biofeedback induced relaxation has been shown to improve lung function.

Massage therapy has a positive effect on children with asthma in several studies. A twenty-minute bedtime backrub by a parent improved lung function after five weeks in children four to eight years of age in one study.

Honey in combination with other substances like nigella sativa (black cumin) or celery seeds improved asthma symptoms. However, honey alone has not been shown to improve asthma symptoms.

Essential oils have not been well studied, and there is no definitive data showing benefit of diffused essential oils in the treatment of asthma. Data does confirm the release of harmful volatile organic compounds from use of lavender, eucalyptus, and tea tree essential oils. Terpenes released from diffused essential oils are associated with nocturnal breathlessness and decreased lung function in asthma.

Acupuncture, a practice thousands of years old, is believed to improve airway flow. Data does not definitively prove this.

Salt room use for treatment of asthma has not been well studied, and there is no data to support its use.

Chiropractic spinal manipulative therapy intervention has shown no benefit over conventional asthma medications in mild to moderate asthma.

Over-the-counter topical vapor rubs and turpentine oil placed on the chest in children can be fatal if ingested.

Sleep Issues – What Should I Know?

How much sleep did you get last night? How many hours of sleep does your child typically get each night? Chances are you and your child are not sleeping enough. When children sleep restfully, they are healthier, learn better, and have fewer behavioral issues. Making sleep a priority is important. So, how many hours of sleep are enough?

- Infants four months to twelve months -twelve to sixteen hours (including naps)
- Toddlers one to two years old -eleven to fourteen hours (including naps)
- Three to five years old – ten to thirteen hours (including naps)
- Six to twelve years old – nine to twelve hours
- Thirteen to eighteen years old – eight to ten hours

Of course, the quantity of sleep is important, but the quality of sleep is often overlooked. Many kids have difficulty falling asleep and poor quality of sleep. Sleep hygiene is the practice of preparing the body for sleep. Kids need to be taught sleep hygiene just like they are trained in hygienic behaviors like handwashing, bathing, and brushing their teeth. The first step to quality sleep is setting a bedtime and being consistent with the schedule. Provide kids with an electronics bedtime.

They should turn off cell phones, tablets, and the TV at least one hour prior to bedtime for restful sleep. Blue light emitted from the screens of our electronic devices prevents the release of melatonin, a natural substance our body makes to induce sleep. Reading a book or listening to soft music are great ways to prepare for sleep. Also, try to eat dinner at least three to four hours prior to bedtime. For older children and teens, they should not exercise within three hours of bedtime, because exercise is an alerting behavior. Kids should avoid eating chocolate or drinking sodas due to the caffeine present. If a child still has difficulty falling asleep despite appropriate sleep hygiene, they should be evaluated for insomnia. In addition, consider a trial of melatonin thirty minutes prior to bedtime. Melatonin is not a prescription and can be purchased over-the-counter. Check with your doctor to determine which brand and dose are best for your child.

Expert Tip

Keeping a daily sleep diary recording your child's bedtime, nighttime routines, and sleep issues is helpful to make a clear assessment of sleep concerns.

Children with asthma frequently have nocturnal symptoms awakening them from sleep. Classically, asthma worsens overnight with episodes of coughing, wheezing, and shortness of breath preventing restful sleep. Controlling asthma symptoms with optimal medications eliminates sleep disruption and daytime sleepiness.

If children snore overnight, gasp, have pauses in their breathing, or awaken for unknown reasons, they may have obstructive sleep apnea (OSA). In Latin "a" means without and "pnea" means breath. Children with OSA have blockage of their airway during sleep causing them to stop breathing or become apneic. Enlarged tonsils sitting at the back of the throat and adenoids in the upper airway are often the cause of airway obstruction. Obesity and elevated body mass index are significant risk factors for the development of OSA. Children have different OSA symptoms than adults. Kids with OSA have symptoms such as hyperactivity, impulsivity, difficulty learning, and behavior issues. They may also wet the bed. A sleep study is used to formally diagnose sleep apnea. During a sleep study, your child will sleep overnight in a sleep lab with continuous monitoring of breathing, heart activity, oxygen level, limb, and brain activity. Sleep studies offer detailed information about your child's sleep. Weight loss helps resolve sleep apnea in some overweight children. For mild OSA, medical treatment includes use of a nasal corticosteroid spray with montelukast to control upper airway inflammation and swelling. For moderate to severe OSA, surgical removal of the adenoids and/or tonsils may be needed. In some children, continuous positive airway pressure (CPAP), a device that blows pressure in the airway through a machine with a mask covering the nose and mouth may be needed to treat OSA.

Restless leg syndrome (RLS) in children can cause difficulty staying asleep. It is a condition characterized by an urge to move the legs and an unpleasant sensation in the legs. A sleep study can be used to diagnose RLS or periodic limb movement disorder, a similar condition. Iron deficiency is associated with RLS, and a blood test can determine if your child will benefit from iron supplementation.

Sleep terrors occur when children awaken suddenly from sleep with a scream, confused, and agitated. Children three to seven years of age are the most likely to suffer from this. Typically sleep or night terrors happen three to four hours after sleep onset. Kids are difficult to soothe during a sleep terror and may not be fully awake during the event. They usually do not remember the sleep terror. If the event happens consistently at the same time each night, consider awakening the child thirty minutes prior to the usual time of the sleep terror. The scheduled awakening may help to shift the sleep cycle and extinguish the sleep terrors.

Sleepwalking is common in children and usually happens in the first third of the night. Children eight to twelve years of age are the most likely to sleepwalk. Safety measures are important to prevent injury. Consider placing a door alarm, floor mat alarm, or motion sensor to alert you that a child has left their room. Safety gates are helpful for stairs in young children.

If your child has excessive daytime sleepiness, they should be assessed for narcolepsy, a neurological condition caused by intrusion of deep sleep or rapid eye movement sleep (REM) into wakefulness. Children with narcolepsy in addition to excessive daytime sleepiness have cataplexy or loss of muscle control with strong emotion, sleep paralysis, and hallucinations. Kids can be diagnosed with this as young as five years of age, and this is usually a lifelong disorder. A diagnosis of narcolepsy is made with a sleep study and multiple sleep latency test (MSLT). During a MSLT, a child takes a series of short naps, and the time it takes to fall asleep is examined. There is no cure for narcolepsy. Children are encouraged to take planned naps during the day. In addition, central nervous system stimulants may be prescribed to decrease sleepiness.

Is COVID-19 Dangerous for Kids with Asthma?

Children are estimated to represent 1-2 percent of the total cases of severe acute respiratory syndrome coronavirus 2 (SARS-CoV-2) infection worldwide. In the United States, cases of coronavirus 2019 (COVID-19) were first reported in children in March of 2020. Per the Centers for Disease Control and Prevention (CDC) website, recent data show children comprise 7.3 percent of all the COVID-19 cases in the United States. The most common symptoms of coronavirus disease (COVID-19) in children are dry cough and fever. Additional symptoms of infection include fatigue, difficulty breathing, diarrhea, vomiting, body ache, loss of taste, loss of smell, sore throat, and poor feeding. Many children may be asymptomatic or have few symptoms. Overall, children have milder symptoms of COVID-19 than adults and lower hospitalizations rates than adults. However, in the US, hospitalization rates in children are rising, with one in three children hospitalized due to COVID-19 admitted to the intensive care unit.

Expert Tip

Use of nebulized medications is not recommended in children and people with COVID-19 due to increased risk of transmission of COVID-19 via aerosolized droplets.

There is not enough evidence to say definitively if children with asthma have worsened outcome with COVID-19. Currently, it is suspected children most at risk for severe infection with COVID-19 are infants less than one year of age and children with underlying medical conditions such as chronic lung disease, uncontrolled asthma, obesity, neurologic/developmental disorders, weakened immune systems, and cardiovascular concerns. Hospitalization rates are higher in kids of Hispanic/Latino descent and non-Hispanic Black children compared with white children. Pediatric hospitals and emergency departments have seen a decline in asthma visits. It is unclear if this is due to improved adherence to asthma regimens during the pandemic or avoidance of medical facilities due to the fear of contracting COVID-19. It is important to follow closely with your doctor to determine how to best control your child's asthma during the pandemic. Wearing a mask, socially distancing, and handwashing are important in preventing the spread of COVID-19 and keeping you and your child healthy.

You may have heard about a complication of COVID-19 in children called multisystem inflammatory syndrome (MIS-C). This occurs in children with SARS-CoV-2 infection who are sick with varied symptoms including fever, diarrhea, vomiting, skin rash, mouth sores, low blood pressure (hypo-tension), and shock, a life-threatening decrease in blood and oxygen to vital organs. Children with MIS-C may have symptoms of rash, red eyes, swollen hands and feet, swollen strawberry-looking tongue, cracked lips, and enlarged neck lymph nodes similar to another condition called Kawasaki disease. With MIS-C, there are usually more than two body organs involved.

Expert Tip

Children with asthma are not considered to be at increased risk of developing MIS-C.

Diagnosis of MIS-C has happened weeks after having COVID-19 or in children with no known COVID-19 infec-tion. However, usually children test positive for SARS-Co-V-2 antibodies. There have been more reported cases of MIS-C in boys than girls, and the majority of children affected are Hispanic or non-Hispanic Blacks. Most patients require hospitalization in the pediatric intensive care unit (PICU) for treatment. MIS-C is treated with supportive care, meaning fluids, intravenous immunoglobulins (IVIG), and steroids. The Centers for Disease Control and Preven-tion (CDC) continues to monitor the reported cases and deaths from MIS-C. This syndrome is a sobering reminder that kids can be severely affected by COVID-19.

In the United States, vaccinations for COVID-19 have recently been approved for use in adults, and for the Pfizer vaccine, in children sixteen years of age and older. Approval for young children has not been granted, but there are clinical trials ongoing for children twelve and older. Make sure you check with your pediatrician regarding what COVID-19 vaccination is best for your child.

Are Face Masks Safe for Children with Asthma?

COVID-19 is spread by aerosolized droplets that can float through the air. We now know that virus particles can spread greater than six feet. Face masks are important protection from the transmission of COVID-19 for children and adults. It is safe for children two years and older to wear face masks. Children younger than two or those who cannot remove a mask independently should not wear a mask. If a child is having difficulty breathing they should also not wear a mask. As a healthcare provider, I wear a face shield and face mask daily. You may consider a face shield for your child if they are unable to keep a mask on their face. Masks for children should have two or more layers, be breathable, and washable. The mask should completely cover a child's nose and mouth. The mask should fit closely to your child's face and should not have large gaps on the sides. Adjustable straps around the ear are helpful to make sure the mask does not slip down. Masks with an exhalation valve or vent allow virus particles to enter and leave with your breath and are not recommended. A cloth face mask or covering will adequately protect your child.

Expert Tip

N95 masks filter out 95 percent of airborne particles including large and small particles when properly fitted over the mouth and nose. They are considered hospital grade and should be worn by medical professionals.

Hospital grade masks such as N95 masks are not needed for children. Make sure that your child keeps their cloth face mask covering the nose and the mouth. Virus particles can enter through the nose, eyes, and mouth. Make sure that you teach your child how to take off their mask. They should remove the mask from the ear loops or straps behind the ears. Remind them not to touch their eyes, nose, or mouth before washing their hands. Children should be taught to wash their hands for at least twenty seconds after taking off the mask. Cloth masks can be washed and dried with your laundry using the hottest possible setting allowed for your clothes and completely dried.

Many of the patients I treat have asked for school exemptions for mask wearing in their child with asthma. Mask recommendations are in place to protect everyone from COVID-19. I recommend children with asthma and all children over two years of age wear a mask when out in public during the COVID-19 pandemic. If they are having difficulty breathing, their asthma medications may need to be adjusted.

Should My Child with Asthma Attend Virtual or In-Person School?

For many children, in-person learning is optimal and home-schooling has been challenging. However, the uncertain risks of COVID-19 transmission and infection when children return to school has created a dilemma for how to best educate and protect kids. Currently, it does not appear that children with mild asthma have increased risk for worsened COVID-19. However, there is not enough information to know this for sure. The decision to homeschool or send your child back to in-person school is a personal one and should also be discussed with your doctor who knows your child's medical history. Currently, for children with uncontrolled asthma or who have had hospitalizations for asthma in the last six months to one year, I recommend homeschool or virtual school. This offers the safest option for children with asthma who may be at higher risk for complications with COVID-19 infection. Another possible option is home-school pods, where small groups of children work with a teacher. This may offer less risk for exposure while maintaining opportunities for socialization. However, for many, a homeschool pod is not an option. Fortunately, most public and private schools offer the option of virtual school, in-person, or a hybrid approach.

Expert Tip

If you opt for brick and mortar school, make sure you understand the measures in place; your school should clean frequently, socially distance, temperature check, and track COVID-19 cases.

The SARS-CoV-2 virus causing COVID-19 infection is spread through aerosolized droplets originating from the upper respiratory tract. When droplets remain suspended in the air, increased risk for indoor transmission is possible. Scientists have speculated about airborne spread of the SARS-CoV-2 virus with air conditioners supporting viral infection; however, this is not proven. Masking, social distancing, changing air conditioner filters regularly, and working in a well-ventilated room minimize any possible risk of airborne spread. The virus can survive on cardboard for twenty-four hours and up to three days on stainless steel and plastic surfaces. It is critical that shared spaces with high touch areas such as light switches, countertops, faucets, bathrooms, and door handles are frequently disinfected.

Does My Child with Asthma Need a Flu Vaccine?

Influenza "the flu" is a contagious respiratory virus that attacks the upper and lower respiratory tract. Influenza can cause mild to severe symptoms including fever, cough, runny nose, sore throat, body aches, and fatigue. Asthma is a risk factor for developing severe complications from the flu including an asthma attack, pneumonia, and respiratory distress requiring hospitalization. Children are more likely to get sick from the flu, with those under five years of age at higher risk for complications. The influenza vaccine is recommended for everyone six months of age and older to protect against severe illness with influenza virus. Yes, that means you and your child with asthma should get the flu vaccine this year. The injectable flu vaccine or flu shot is safe and effective for children six months of age and older. The nasal spray flu vaccine is not recommended for children two to four years of age who have asthma or a history of wheezing in the past twelve months. If your child is younger than six months, you should obtain the flu vaccine to protect your infant from infection.

Expert Tip

You cannot get the flu from the flu vaccine. People who got sick after the flu vaccine may have infection from another virus or have been exposed to the flu before they got their flu vaccine.

There are two major flu viruses, influenza A and influenza B. Every year, there are small changes in the surface proteins of the influenza virus. The flu vaccine targets these surface proteins. A new flu vaccine is manufactured each year with the three to four influenza virus strains predicted to be circulating in the upcoming year. That is why you need to get a new flu vaccine every year when flu season starts. The benefits of taking the flu vaccine are clear; you can reduce the risk of having to go to the doctor by 40-60 percent and reduce hospitalization risk for children. When you get the flu vaccine you protect those around you. Make sure you speak with your doctor about which flu vaccine is best. There are several available on the market. This year more than ever a flu vaccine is important for kids with asthma to protect against serious complications from the flu that may make children more susceptible to COVID-19.

Day Care, Wheezing, and Asthma – Is There a Connection?

When infants and young children attend day care or school for the first time, they develop recurrent illness as they are exposed to new viruses. Children may be sick every three to four weeks, making the first year in day care stressful. Wheezing, or whistling of the airway caused by constriction of the airway muscle, in children is common with a prevalence or occurrence rate of up to 40 percent. Young children wheeze because their airway tubes are smaller and collapse more easily with exhalation. There is a strong connection between viral bronchiolitis, infection of the small airway tubes, and recurrent wheezing. However, most young children who wheeze will not go on to develop asthma. In fact, the risk of developing asthma in young children who wheeze has been well studied. There are certain factors increasing the probability of wheezing with asthma. Specifically, children are higher risk for asthma if they wheeze in addition to having parental asthma, doctor diagnosed eczema, or environmental or food allergen sensitivity. If none of these risk factors are present, there is a high chance your child will not go on to become asthmatic. All children who wheeze will benefit from a trial of a rescue medication like albuterol. This medication quickly opens the airway by loosening the airway muscle. Young children who have recurrent episodes of bronchiolitis requiring hospitalization should be considered for a trial of inhaled corticosteroids and asthma management. Improvement with asthma medications and worsening off of treatment assist with diagnosis of asthma in young children since routine lung function testing cannot be completed.

Why Are There Disparities in Asthma Outcomes?

Differences in health outcomes are correlated with health disparities or a higher burden of illness, disability, injury, or death experienced by one group relative to another. The major health outcome disparity or difference with asthma is that it affects children disproportionately more than adults. However, as a pediatric pulmonologist and lifelong asthmatic, it is obvious to me that all children with asthma do not have the same outcome, even when prescribed the same medications. Presumably, when children take the same medicine for the same condition, there should be the same outcome, right? Unfortunately, this is not the case. One size does not fit all when it comes to who suffers from asthma. The question from doctors, scientists, kids, and parents alike is, why? The answer is a complex comingling of factors such as socioeconomic status, race, gender, ethnicity, genetics, and bias.

With asthma there are clear health disparities related to gender. Before puberty, boys are more likely than girls to have asthma and to be hospitalized for an asthma exacerbation. After puberty, asthma is more common in girls. In fact, during adolescence, there is a decline in the severity of asthma illness in males compared to females. For girls, early menstruation is associated with a significantly increased odds of asthma in some studies.

More complex are the disparities in asthma outcomes correlated with race, ethnicity, and socioeconomic status. Some of the differences in outcome for children are centered around how children of different backgrounds are treated by doctors. Physician bias has been documented in asthma care. Minority children are less likely to be prescribed a controller medication when indicated, and minority families are also less likely to take the medication when prescribed. Black children with asthma are less likely to have a written asthma treatment plan and in one study were shown to have fewer visits with their doctors.

Expert Tip

As a parent or caregiver of an asthmatic, it is important that you are educated about asthma and understand the importance of giving medications when appropriate. You should feel empowered to ask your doctor questions about the medications prescribed to review any concerns or reservations you have about a medication.

There has not always been a large difference in the rates of asthma between Black and white children. The prevalence of asthma was similar in white and Black children from the early 1980s to the mid-1990s. However, in the 2000s, the rates of asthma in minority children exploded. Currently, children in the US who are racial and ethnic minorities are more likely to have worsened asthma illness, more frequent emergency department visits, hospitalizations, and death from asthma. In the US, the rates of asthma in Black children are significantly higher than white children across all income levels. Emergency department and urgent care visits are highest among Black children under four years old. Studies show African American children have an almost fivefold higher asthma mortality or death rate when compared to non-Hispanic_white children. Hispanic children are two times more likely to visit the emergency department and one and a half times more likely to die due to asthma compared with non-Hispanic white children. These trends are disturbing, and the underlying reasons for these statistics are related in part to access to care. Children of ethnic minorities are more likely to have limited access to primary care and subspecialists.

Pollution and environmental exposures are triggers for asthma. Studies have shown increased risk for asthma with closer proximity to a highway or large road. The legacy of housing discrimination called redlining (practice of mortgage lenders refusing mortgage loans in certain areas based upon race) translates into African Americans living in less desirable locations by factories and roads, contributing to an increased burden of disease. Asthma has also been linked to poor housing quality. Home ownership is associated with a lower risk of having a child with asthma. Minorities own homes in lower numbers than their white counterparts.

The latest data from the CDC shows the prevalence of childhood asthma in the US is highest in non-Hispanic Blacks, followed by Puerto Ricans, with Mexican Americans having the lowest numbers. Ethnicity is thought to play a role in the severity of asthma. African ancestry is associated with reduced lung function and increased risk for asthma in African Americans and Puerto Ricans. The difference in asthma prevalence between Puerto Ricans and Mexican Americans may be due to the African versus Native American ancestry found in these respective groups. Mexican Americans have Native American ancestry, associated with higher FEV1 or lung function.

The racial and ethnic implications for asthma disparities do not account for all differences seen in kids. Poverty can affect asthma outcomes independent of race and ethnicity. The reasons for this are multifactorial and not fully understood. Fortunately, scientists and doctors continue to study disparities in asthma outcomes. As a parent or caregiver or a child with asthma, awareness of health disparities in asthma is important and a step toward trying to eliminate them.

Does Being Overweight Affect Childhood Asthma?

There is a childhood obesity epidemic in the US with roughly one in five children considered obese. Kids are more sedentary, playing video games, and not going outside to play. COVID-19 restrictions and fears have magnified many of the risk factors for obesity in children. Obesity is defined as a body mass index (BMI) greater than or equal to the ninety-fifth percentile and overweight is a BMI from the eighty-fifth to ninety-fourth percentile. Body mass index is calculated by dividing your child's weight in kg by height squared. Your doctor can review your child's height, weight, and BMI with you at your next office visit.

For many years, the numbers of children with asthma and obesity have risen together, but until recently, it was unclear if the two were related in children. A new study has shown obesity is directly related to risk for asthma, and reducing obesity will likely reduce asthma prevalence.

Obese children with asthma have reduced response to inhaled corticosteroids making their asthma more difficult to control. The exact reasons for this are not known, but some reported explanations include altered lung function with obesity, increased risk for reflux, hormonal changes, and systemic inflammation seen with obesity. Obesity has been associated with depression. For some children, they may be less likely to follow through with use of their asthma medications due to depression.

Some children who are obese do not have asthma, although they have shortness of breath with activity. Cardiopulmonary exercise testing (CPET) evaluates heart, lung, and metabolic effort to determine the origin of difficulty breathing. During testing, children perform vigorous activity while heart and lung function are measured. Children with and without asthma may report difficulty breathing because they are not used to exercising or deconditioned. As they become more comfortable and fit, their breathlessness with exercise should improve. CPET is important to help differentiate if a child has a heart issue or asthma.

Diets are not recommended for any children. Instead, healthy eating choices and more movement should be encouraged to control weight symptoms. Children should exercise for at least thirty minutes five days per week. Exercise can be dancing, a video game with movement, or an organized team sport. Most importantly, it should be fun. Kids with asthma can exercise safely with the right medications.

Children can do something we as adults cannot—grow taller. As they grow and stretch out, this will help resolve some of their weight concerns. Make sure you speak with your pediatrician about how to help your child achieve a healthy weight. Teaching them healthy eating and exercise habits while they are young is important and useful for a lifetime.

Is This Anxiety or Asthma?

Difficulty breathing produces anxiety and depression in many patients with asthma. It makes sense that when a child has a hard time breathing and symptoms are unpredictable, they may be scared and worried. Children may also have anxiety that worsens their asthma symptoms. Alternatively, there are kids who do not have asthma, and their shortness of breath is purely due to anxiety. Children with anxiety and/or depression should be evaluated by a behavioral pediatrician, psychologist, or psychiatrist to determine if treatment with therapy or medicines is needed. Breathing tests are helpful for children over five years of age to distinguish if a child has asthma and/or anxiety.

Can Breathing Techniques Improve Asthma in Children?

In children, breathing exercises have not been proven to assist with asthma symptoms when used alone and should never be a substitute for taking asthma medications. There are a number of breathing techniques practiced by adults with asthma. However, young children often have difficulty coordinating their breathing. For older children, there may be some benefit in working with a speech therapist if a child has asthma and anxiety or vocal cord dysfunction. Pursed lip breathing involves breathing in through your nose with your mouth closed. Kids should breathe deeply and try to fill their lungs over one to two seconds and then blow out through their mouth with pursed (puckered) lips. The exhalation (breath out) should be for twice as long as the inhalation (breath in), or two to four seconds. This breathing method may assist with controlling shortness of breath by keeping the airway open for longer and releasing trapped air in the lungs. It also promotes relaxation. Keep in mind, asthma cannot be controlled with breathing exercises, and medications are how asthma is treated.

The Road Ahead

Take a deep breath and feel empowered. You now understand the basics of breathing and the details of asthma. This book has given you a roadmap to successful treatment of asthma in children. As a parent or caregiver of a child with asthma, you are now better prepared for the journey ahead. I wish you and your child health and happiness as you work together with your doctor to create a successful asthma care plan meeting your child's specific needs.

References

1. A report from the National Asthma Education and Prevention Program Coordinating Committee Expert Panel Working Group. 2020 Focused Updates to The Asthma Management Guidelines. National Heart, Lung, and Blood Institute, National Institutes of Health; 2020. Available from: www.nhlbi.nih.gov. Accessed January 9, 2021.

2. Abbas AS, Ghozy S, Minh LHN, Hashan MR, Soliman AL, Van NT, Hirayama K, Huy NT. Honey in Bronchial Asthma: From Folk Tales to Scientific Facts. J Med Food. 2019 Jun;22(6):543-550. doi: 10.1089/jmf.2018.4303. Epub 2019 May 24. PMID: 31135254.

3. Adkins SH, Anderson KN, Goodman AB, Twentyman E, Danielson ML, Kimball A, Click ES, Ko JY, Evans ME, Weissman DN, Melstrom P, Kiernan E, Krishnasamy V, Rose DA, Jones CM, King BA, Ellington SR, Pollack LA, Wiltz JL; Lung Injury Clinical Task Force and the Lung Injury Epidemiology/Surveillance Task Force. Demographics, Substance Use Behaviors, and Clinical Characteristics of Adolescents With e-Cigarette, or Vaping, Product Use-Associated Lung Injury (EVALI) in the United States in 2019. JAMA Pediatr. 2020 Jul 1;174(7):e200756. doi: 10.1001/jamapediatrics.2020.0756. Epub 2020 Jul 6. PMID: 32421164; PMCID: PMC7235914.

4. Aggarwal B, Mulgirigama A, Berend N. Exercise-induced bronchoconstriction: prevalence, pathophysiology, patient impact, diagnosis and management. NPJ Prim Care Respir Med. 2018 Aug 14;28(1):31. doi: 10.1038/s41533-018-0098-2. PMID: 30108224; PMCID: PMC6092370.

5. Akinbami LJ, Simon AE, Rossen LM. Changing Trends in Asthma Prevalence Among Children. Pediatrics. 2016 Jan;137(1):1–7. doi: 10.1542/peds.2015-2354. Epub 2015 Dec 28. PMID: 26712860; PMCID: PMC4755484.

6. Bowatte G, Lodge C, Lowe AJ, Erbas B, Perret J, Abramson MJ, Matheson M, Dharmage SC. The influence of childhood traffic-related air pollution exposure on asthma, allergy and sensitization: a systematic review and a meta-analysis of birth cohort studies. Allergy. 2015 Mar;70(3):245-56. doi: 10.1111/all.12561. Epub 2014 Dec 31. PMID: 25495759.

7. Castro-Rodriguez JA, Forno E, Rodriguez-Martinez CE, Celedón JC. Risk and Protective Factors for Childhood Asthma: What Is the Evidence? J Allergy Clin Immunol Pract. 2016 Nov-Dec;4(6):1111-1122. doi: 10.1016/j.jaip.2016.05.003. Epub 2016 Jun 8. PMID: 27286779; PMCID: PMC5107168.

8. Castro-Rodríguez JA, Holberg CJ, Wright AL, Martinez FD. A clinical index to define risk of asthma in young children with recurrent wheezing. Am J Respir Crit

Care Med. 2000 Oct;162(4 Pt 1):1403-6. doi: 10.1164/ajrccm.162.4.9912111. PMID: 11029352.

9. Chan CK, Kuo ML, Shen JJ, See LC, Chang HH, Huang JL. Ding Chuan Tang, a Chinese herb decoction, could improve airway hyper-responsiveness in stabilized asthmatic children: a randomized, double-blind clinical trial. Pediatr Allergy Immunol. 2006 Aug;17(5):316-22. doi: 10.1111/j.1399-3038.2006.00406.x. PMID: 16846448.

10. Collaco JM, McGrath-Morrow SA. Respiratory Phenotypes for Preterm Infants, Children, and Adults: Bronchopulmonary Dysplasia and More. Ann Am Thorac Soc. 2018 May;15(5):530-538. doi: 10.1513/AnnalsATS.201709-756FR. PMID: 29328889.

11. Del Giacco SR, Firinu D, Bjermer L, Carlsen KH. Exercise and asthma: an overview. Eur Clin Respir J. 2015 Nov 3;2:27984. doi: 10.3402/ecrj.v2.27984. PMID: 26672959; PMCID: PMC4653278.

12. Ege MJ, Mayer M, Normand AC, Genuneit J, Cookson WO, Braun-Fahrländer C, Heederik D, Piarroux R, von Mutius E; GABRIELA Transregio 22 Study Group. Exposure to environmental microorganisms and childhood asthma. N Engl J Med. 2011 Feb 24;364(8):701-9. doi: 10.1056/NEJMoa1007302. PMID: 21345099.

13. Fuseini H, Newcomb DC. Mechanisms Driving Gender Differences in Asthma. Curr Allergy Asthma Rep. 2017 Mar;17(3):19. doi: 10.1007/s11882-017-0686-1. PMID: 28332107; PMCID: PMC5629917.

14. Global Initiative for Asthma (GINA). Global strategy for asthma management and prevention (Updated 2020). Available from: www.ginasthma.org. Accessed January 9, 2021.

15. Hughes HK, Matsui EC, Tschudy MM, Pollack CE, Keet CA. Pediatric Asthma Health Disparities: Race, Hardship, Housing, and Asthma in a National Survey. Acad Pediatr. 2017 Mar;17(2):127-134. doi: 10.1016/j.acap.2016.11.011. Epub 2016 Nov 19. PMID: 27876585; PMCID: PMC5337434.

16. Kuruvilla ME, Lee FE, Lee GB. Understanding Asthma Phenotypes, Endotypes, and Mechanisms of Disease. Clin Rev Allergy Immunol. 2019 Apr;56(2):219-233. doi: 10.1007/s12016-018-8712-1. PMID: 30206782; PMCID: PMC6411459.

17. Lang JE, Bunnell HT, Hossain MJ, Wysocki T, Lima JJ, Finkel TH, Bacharier L, Dempsey A, Sarzynski L, Test M, Forrest CB. Being Overweight or Obese and the Development of Asthma. Pediatrics. 2018 Dec;142(6):e20182119. doi: 10.1542/peds.2018-2119. PMID: 30478238.

18. Milner JD, Stein DM, McCarter R, Moon RY. Early infant multivitamin supplementation is associated with increased risk for food allergy and asthma. Pediatrics. 2004 Jul;114(1):27-32. doi: 10.1542/peds.114.1.27. PMID: 15231904.

19. Na'ara S, Vainer I, Amit M, Gordin A. Foreign Body Aspiration in Infants and Older Children: A Comparative Study. Ear Nose Throat J. 2020 Jan;99(1):47-51. doi: 10.1177/0145561319839900. Epub 2019 Apr 11. PMID: 30974996.

20. National Asthma Education and Prevention Program. *Expert Panel Report 3: Guidelines for the Diagnosis and Management of Asthma.* Bethesda, Maryland: National Heart, Lung, and Blood Institute, National Institutes of Health; 2007.

21. Center for Disease Control and Prevention, "Most Recent National Asthma Data: National Center for Environmental Health," https://www.cdc.gov/asthma/most_recent_national_asthma_data.htm. Accessed January 9, 2021.

22. Pagtakhan RD, Bjelland JC, Landau LI, Loughlin G, Kaltenborn W, Seeley G, Taussig LM. Sex differences in growth patterns of the airways and lung parenchyma in children. J Appl Physiol Respir Environ Exerc Physiol. 1984 May;56(5):1204-10. doi: 10.1152/jappl.1984.56.5.1204. PMID: 6725083.

23. Paruthi S, Brooks LJ, D'Ambrosio C, Hall WA, Kotagal S, Lloyd RM, Malow BA, Maski K, Nichols C, Quan SF, Rosen CL, Troester MM, Wise MS. Consensus Statement of the American Academy of Sleep Medicine on the Recommended Amount of Sleep for Healthy Children: Methodology and Discussion. J Clin Sleep Med.

2016 Nov 15;12(11):1549-1561. doi: 10.5664/jcsm.6288. PMID: 27707447; PMCID: PMC5078711.

24. Pino-Yanes M, Thakur N, Gignoux CR, Galanter JM, Roth LA, Eng C, Nishimura KK, Oh SS, Vora H, Huntsman S, Nguyen EA, Hu D, Drake KA, Conti DV, Moreno-Estrada A, Sandoval K, Winkler CA, Borrell LN, Lurmann F, Islam TS, Davis A, Farber HJ, Meade K, Avila PC, Serebrisky D, Bibbins-Domingo K, Lenoir MA, Ford JG, Brigino-Buenaventura E, Rodriguez-Cintron W, Thyne SM, Sen S, Rodriguez-Santana JR, Bustamante CD, Williams LK, Gilliland FD, Gauderman WJ, Kumar R, Torgerson DG, Burchard EG. Genetic ancestry influences asthma susceptibility and lung function among Latinos. J Allergy Clin Immunol. 2015 Jan;135(1):228-35. doi: 10.1016/j.jaci.2014.07.053. Epub 2014 Oct 6. PMID: 25301036; PMCID: PMC4289103.

25. Sherman CB, Tosteson TD, Tager IB, Speizer FE, Weiss ST. Early childhood predictors of asthma. Am J Epidemiol. 1990 Jul;132(1):83-95. doi: 10.1093/oxfordjournals.aje.a115646. PMID: 2356817.

26. Taussig LM, Wright AL, Holberg CJ, Halonen M, Morgan WJ, Martinez FD. Tucson Children's Respiratory Study: 1980 to present. J Allergy Clin Immunol. 2003 Apr;111(4):661-75; quiz 676. doi: 10.1067/mai.2003.162. PMID: 12704342.

27. Valerio MA, Andreski PM, Schoeni RF, McGonagle KA. Examining the association between childhood asthma

and parent and grandparent asthma status: implications for practice. Clin Pediatr (Phila). 2010 Jun;49(6):535-41. doi: 10.1177/0009922809356465. PMID: 20507869; PMCID: PMC3020897.

28. van der Hulst AE, Klip H, Brand PL. Risk of developing asthma in young children with atopic eczema: a systematic review. J Allergy Clin Immunol. 2007 Sep;120(3):565-9. doi: 10.1016/j.jaci.2007.05.042. Epub 2007 Jul 26. PMID: 17655920.

29. von Mutius E, Smits HH. Primary prevention of asthma: from risk and protective factors to targeted strategies for prevention. Lancet. 2020 Sep 19;396(10254):854-866. doi: 10.1016/S0140-6736(20)31861-4. Epub 2020 Sep 7. PMID: 32910907.

30. Willett JG, Bennett M, Hair EC, Xiao H, Greenberg MS, Harvey E, Cantrell J, Vallone D. Recognition, use and perceptions of JUUL among youth and young adults. Tob Control. 2019 Jan;28(1):115-116. doi: 10.1136/tobaccocontrol-2018-054273. Epub 2018 Apr 18. PMID: 29669749.

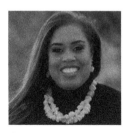

Joi S. Lucas, MD, is a board-certified pediatric pulmonologist and pediatrician in Orlando and Lakeland, Florida. She is the Chief of Pediatrics at Lakeland Regional Health. It is her goal to empower children with asthma and their families to be healthier and thrive by offering innovative products and educational tools focused on improving the quality of life for asthmatics.

After attending Spelman College in Atlanta, Georgia, Dr. Lucas graduated from Howard University College of Medicine, following in her mother's footsteps some thirty years later. She completed a residency in Pediatrics at Orlando Health Arnold Palmer Hospital for Children, and a Pediatric Pulmonology Fellowship at Children's National Medical Center in Washington, DC. Dr. Lucas is a member of several local and national medical organizations and Alpha Kappa Alpha Sorority, Incorporated. In her free time, she loves to travel, go to the beach, spend time with her family and friends. She also enjoys volunteering with children's charities in Florida.

Learn more at www.theasthmabook.com

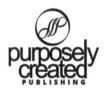

CREATING DISTINCTIVE BOOKS
WITH INTENTIONAL RESULTS

We're a collaborative group of creative masterminds
with a mission to produce high-quality books to position
you for monumental success in the marketplace.

Our professional team of writers, editors, designers,
and marketing strategists work closely together to ensure
that every detail of your book is a clear representation
of the message in your writing.

Want to know more?
Write to us at info@publishyourgift.com
or call (888) 949-6228

Discover great books, exclusive offers, and more at
www.PublishYourGift.com

Connect with us on social media

@publishyourgift

CPSIA information can be obtained
at www.ICGtesting.com
Printed in the USA
LVHW071621260921
698753LV00023B/1241